Beer

for Your Health

Joe Urbach

www.gardeningaustin.com

www.phytonutrientfarms.com

A

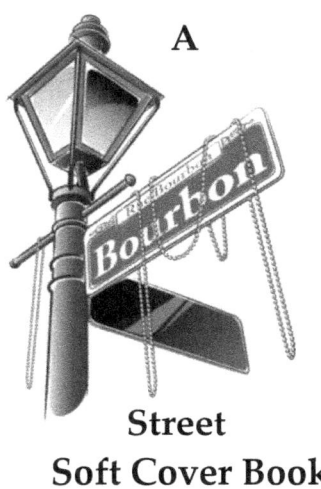

Street
Soft Cover Book

1st published in the United State in 2017 by
Bond Street Publications, a Hojo Enterprises Company

1st Printing 2017

Copyright © Joseph Urbach 2017

All rights reserved under International and Pan-American Copyright Conventions.

DEDICATION

For my Uncle Bob Moyer, with
whom I shared good times and good
beer – here's to more of both!

This book was also written for all of
us who simply want to sit back and
enjoy the occasional cold beer
while we watch the big game, or
cook on the grill, or whatever! The
idea was to give us another reason
to knock back a few brewskies!

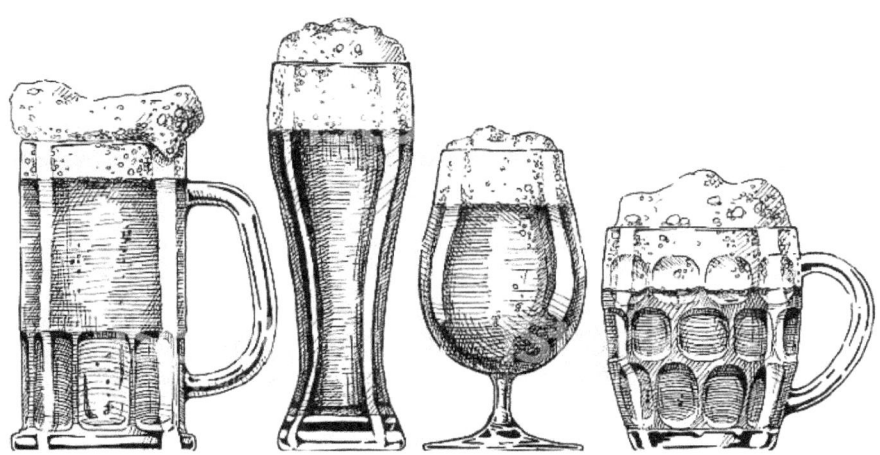

CONTENTS

Forward

Guess what? I am not a scientist, nor a medical doctor, nor a nutritionist, nor any other kind of healthcare worker. I am not a research professional nor have I ever been involved in medical research of any kind. Why do I tell you this? Because it is important that you understand where I am coming from when I present the information that follows. So, please understand that I am not a doctor, I am a gardener, a father, a grandfather, and a diabetic. All of this led me to my concern about nutrition, and in turn, led me on a quest that eventually led to the writing of my ***Phytonutrient Gardening*** series, which was recently rebranded as my ***Yes, Food IS Medicine*** series of books – that then led to my researching the history and health benefits of a great many foods, drinks, and other items, all of which led to this book!

My journey of exploration has convinced me that there is a very serious problem with the fruit and vegetables that are finding their way into our local markets and eventually on to our dinner plates, and that there is a serious problem with our understanding of how what we consume can impact our health. The real concern is that it can quickly impact our health both for good and ill, but we do not seem to understand this.

A doctor I know once told me that he never gave the link between eating and health much thought, "After all," he said, "if it was so important they would have taught it to me in medical school." Sadly, it is important and they don't teach it!

So, like many of you, I set off in search of helpful health information – but alas, most of what I found was of little merit and even less use. I found misinformation, false information and outright lies. Much of the worst of the 'garbage' info I found concerned chocolate, beer, and wine – three of my favorite things - and so this book was

just begging to be written! The information I present in this work is provided for your consideration only and I absolutely do not condone, endorse, or recommend that you take up drinking alcohol or stuffing yourself with candy bars, or even change any of your diet or exercise habits without first consulting your healthcare professional.

My honest belief is that knowledge is power and my goal is to empower **you** with the information that follows so that **you** and your doctor can choose the best course of action for **you** to take to help **you** achieve a better, healthier, happier, and longer life! See the word 'you' in bold so many times? That is because to benefit from the information presented in this book **you** must do this for **yourself**. **You** must read and absorb the info and then **you** must consciously choose how to use it for **your** benefit! No one else can do that for **you**!

Let me say right up front at the beginning of this book that too much of a good thing is not a good thing! Increased alcohol consumption over time will not lead to better health but could, in fact, ruin your health. Moderation is the key word here! Keep that in mind as you read on.

INTRODUCTION

On a hot summer's day, after I have labored to push my lawn mower all over my yard, emptied the grass catcher into the compost bin (over and over again) and cleaned and put away my mower, nothing is a satisfying as relaxing with my favorite ice-cold beer and admiring my yard handiwork. Add a Philadelphia-style soft pretzel to the scene and you will reach nirvana!

But thanks to the so-called beer belly, beer has gotten a reputation as a "bad-for-you" beverage. I am sure each of you has heard, as I so often did, that beer is basically evil and from a health standpoint should always be avoided. "It's not good for you." Well the more research I did into food and drink and how they relate to our health and nutrition the more I discovered the truth, and that is that the thought that any food or drink is fundamentally 'bad' for us is just plain hogwash!

It is time to call BS on that old myth!

Sometimes, nothing but a cold glass of beer will do, especially when you're at the game or visiting your neighbourhood pub with friends. But can sipping a pint be part of a healthy lifestyle?

"There's a strong association between beer and the beer belly, so people automatically assume that beer is fattening or unhealthy," says beer sommelier Mirella Amato, who specializes in the selection and service of ales. "But that's just not true.'"

Shocking, isn't it? But consider this: Beer is fat-free, cholesterol-free and low in carbohydrates. A 341-mL (about 12 ounce) bottle of beer with 5 percent alcohol has 5g of carbohydrates, while a pear with the skin on has 26g.

Now I am not saying you should trade your fruits and veggies in for a steady diet of suds, but enjoying beer in moderation can actually be a healthier beverage choice than soda or sugary fruit cocktails. "Picking beer over another beverage if you're counting your calories is often wise," says Amato.

Beer is not only inherently healthy, it does in fact, offer many health benefits, when consumed in moderation, that the human body truly requires! Moderation in our consumption and enjoyment of this ancient beverage, as with so much in life, is the real key. So, the simple truth is that, enjoyed responsibly, beer can actually be a healthy drink choice. But how much is considered moderate and how much is too much? How has this drink, that has been a favorite of all classes of man, from farm hand to pharaoh, influenced mankind throughout history? How has it grown and evolved in its history? Just what benefits does beer have to offer us?

I set out to answer those questions and more when I first started this book. I had just published a book on the history and health benefits of coffee, ___Let's get Coffee___ and one on wine and chocolate, ___Wine, Chocolate, and Your Good Health___, (both currently available at Amazon.com and bookstores everywhere) and I knew form writing those two books that answering the questions I set out above was going to open up many more questions and some surprising answers! I was right! I hope you enjoy reading this book as much as I enjoyed writing it!

Bottoms up!

1. Beer in Ancient History

The Finnish epic Kalevala, collected in written form in the 19th century but based on oral traditions many centuries older, devotes more lines to the origin of beer and brewing than it does to the origin of mankind. Which, I believe, demonstrates the importance mankind has placed on beer and beer brewing, throughout our history.

The British drinking song "Beer, Beer Beer" attributes the invention of beer to the presumably fictional Charlie Mopps:

A long time ago, way back in history
When all there was to drink was nothin' but cups of tea,
Along came a man by the name of Charlie Mopps
And he invented the wonderful drink, and he made it out of hops.

I seriously doubt the truth of the lyrics but again, it simply demonstrates that we human beings think very highly of this golden brew we call beer. In fact, Beer is one of the oldest beverages humans have produced, dating back to at least the fifth millennium BC and recorded in the written history of ancient Egypt and Mesopotamia and was spread throughout world. Many Historians speculate that prehistoric nomads may have made beer from grain & water before even learning to make bread. It may well have been the desire of our hunter gatherer ancestors to brew beer that led

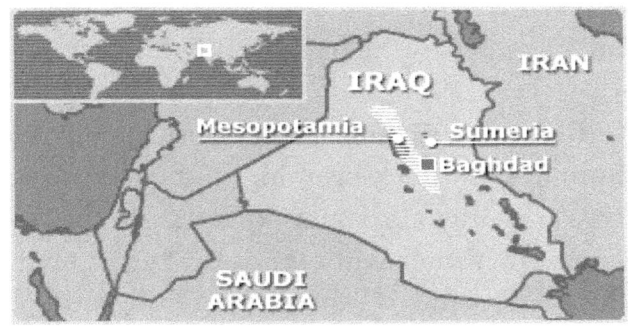

them to settle down in a single location and begin to farm. Many believe that the desire to brew beer changed the world!

The intoxicant known in English as `beer' takes its name from the Latin `bibere' (by way of the German `bier') meaning `to drink' and the Spanish word for beer, cerveza' comes from the Latin word `cerevisia' for `of beer', giving some indication of the long span human beings have been enjoying the drink. Even so, beer brewing did not originate with the Romans but began many thousands of years earlier.

The first beer in the world was brewed by the ancient Chinese around the year 7000 BC (it was known as *kui*). In the west, however, the process now recognized as beer brewing began in the area of Mesopotamia at the Godin Tepe settlement now in modern-day Iran between 3500 - 3100 BC. Evidence of beer manufacture has been confirmed between these dates but it is probable that the brewing of beer in Sumer (southern Mesopotamia, modern-day Iraq) was in practice much earlier. Some evidence has been interpreted, however, which sets the date of beer brewing at Godin Tepe as early as 10,000 BC when agriculture first developed in the region. While some scholars have contended that beer preceded bread as a staple, it is more likely that beer was `discovered' through grains used for bread-making which accidently fermented.

Beer brewing and drinking are activities that have been part of the human experience seemingly since the dawn of civilization. Around 10,000 years ago, mankind began to move away from living life as nomadic hunter gatherers, and began settling down in one spot to farm the land. Grain, a vital ingredient in beer making, was cultivated by these new agricultural societies.

Beer in Ancient China

A Delaware brewer with a penchant for exotic drinks recently concocted a beer similar to one brewed in China some 9,000 years ago, Sam Calagione, of the Dogfish Head brewery in Rehoboth Beach, Delaware, used a recipe that included rice, honey, and grape and hawthorn fruits. He got the formula from archaeologists who derived it from the residues of pottery jars found in the late Stone Age village of Jiahu in northern China.

The residues are the earliest direct evidence of brewed beverages in ancient China. "We can't prove that an alcoholic beverage was definitely produced in the jars—the alcohol is gone—but it's not that difficult to infer," said Patrick McGovern, an archaeo-chemist at the University of Pennsylvania's Museum of Archaeology and Anthropology in Philadelphia.

McGovern, who is known as the "Indiana Jones" of ancient fermented beverages and an expert in the origins and history of alcoholic beverages, performed the chemical analysis on the pottery. He said fruit juices and liquid honey in a temperate climate would easily ferment, allowing for the production of alcohol.

In addition, he said, the setting of the Jiahu site suggests the pottery jugs likely held alcoholic beverages drunk at funeral or religious ceremonies. Archaeologists uncovered ancient "beer-making tool kits" in underground rooms built between 3400 and 2900 B.C. Discovered at a dig site in the Central Plain of China, the kits included funnels, pots and specialized jugs. The shapes of the objects suggest they could be used for brewing, filtration and storage.

It's the oldest beer-making facility ever discovered in China, and the evidence indicates that these early brewers were already using specialized tools and advanced beer-making techniques.

For instance, the scientists found a pottery stove, which the ancient brewers would have heated to break down carbohydrates to sugar. And the brewery's underground location was important for both storing beer and controlling temperature, too much heat can destroy the enzymes responsible for that carb-to-sugar conversion.

The research group inspected the pots and jugs and found ancient grains that had lingered inside. The grains showed evidence that they had been damaged by malting and mashing, two key steps in beer-making. Residue from inside the uncovered pots and funnels was tested with ion chromatography to find out what the ancient beer was made of. The 5,000-year-old beer "recipe" was published in the journal *Proceedings of the National Academy of Sciences*.

The recipe included a mix of fermented grains: broomcorn millet, barley and Job's tears, a chewy Asian grain also known as Chinese pearl barley. The recipe also called for tubers, the starchy and sugary parts of plants, which were added to sweeten and flavor the beer, the researchers write.

So, what did this ancient beer taste like? The researcher leading the study, Jiajing Wang, an archaeologist from Stanford University, guessed "it would taste a bit sour and a bit sweet."

Finding evidence of barley in the beer was surprising to the scientists. Scientists had never seen barley in China this early before. Although barley is now common throughout China, no one completely understands when and why it first made its way there.

Maybe it was about beer. As Wang said in an email: "Barley was one of the main ingredients for beer brewing in other parts of the world, such as ancient Egypt. It is possible that when barley was introduced from Western Eurasia into the Central Plain of China, it came with the knowledge that the crop was a good ingredient for beer brewing. So, it was not only the introduction of a new crop, but also the movement of knowledge associated with the crop."

McGovern says the new findings show that the Chinese became brew masters early on: They were making barley beer in the same period as "the earliest chemically attested barley beer from Iran" and the "earliest beer-mashing facilities in Egypt," as well as "the earliest wine-making facility in Armenia," he writes in an email.

You don't need a scientist to tell you that beer can be an important part of fostering social relationships. (Think happy hour.) Wang and her co-authors propose that beer production and consumption may have helped shaped the hierarchical societies in the Central Plain of China thousands of years ago. As McGovern notes, it would have been "an exotic ingredient" that elites could have used to impress their friends and stay in power — "much like when we serve up that $70,000 bottle of 1982 Pétrus from Bordeaux" today.

McGovern's findings were published in the journal *Proceedings of the National Academy of Sciences* in December 2004.

In earlier research McGovern found evidence of a similar alcoholic beverage in a 2,700-year-old royal tomb in Turkey—

perhaps that of King Midas. He then collaborated with Calagione, Dogfish Head's president, to re-create the drink.

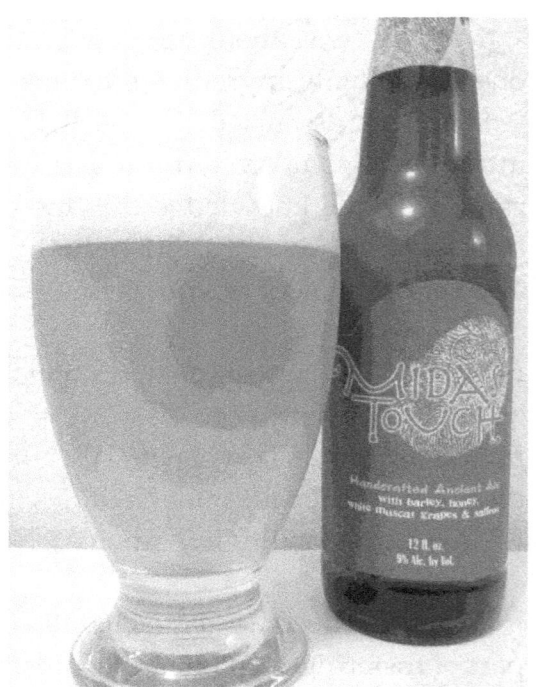

The result was Midas Touch Golden Elixir, a brew that "put us on the map for historical beers," Calagione said. Based on the success of Midas Touch—it has won several beer-festival medals—McGovern again turned to Dogfish Head to brew up the ancient concoction from China. "Hence Chateau Jiahu," Calagione said, referring to the new-old brew's brand name.

Mike Gerhart, distillery manager at Dogfish Head's brewery in Milton, Delaware, led the Chateau Jiahu project. "It was one of the more creative and exciting projects I've ever worked on," he said. McGovern, the archeo-chemist, knew the ingredients of the ancient drink from Jiahu, "but he wasn't sure how to use them or how they would go into action," Gerhart said.

The trick for Gerhart was to mimic the brewing process used in China 9,000 years ago. To get the fermentation started, McGovern imported a mold cake—traditionally used in making Chinese rice wines—from a colleague in Beijing. Gerhart mashed the cake into the rice. Once that became "funky and began to grow," he added other

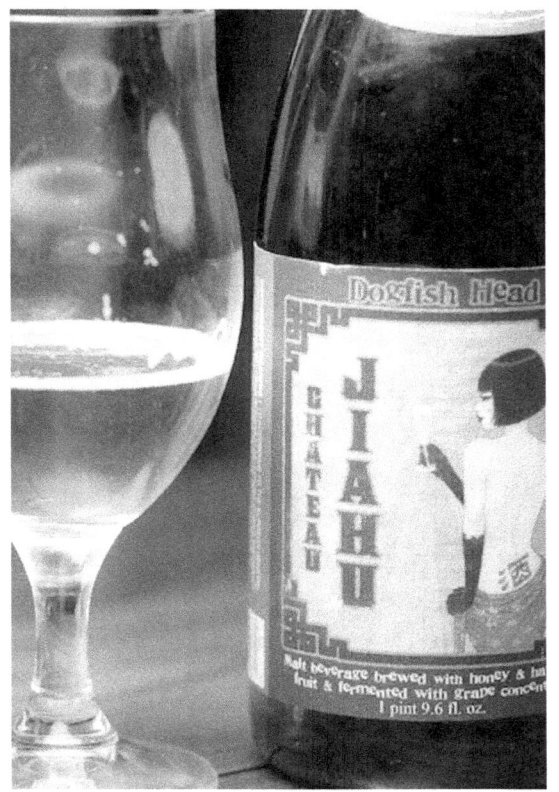

ingredients, including water, honey, grapes, hawthorn fruit, and chrysanthemum flowers.

"We also turned up the brew kettle much higher than we ever would today — we know back then they would have had some type of earthen pot with a fire burning directly below it — to replicate those flavors we know formed, somewhat burnt and caramelized," he said.

To comply with U.S. federal brewing regulations, Gerhart had to add barley malt, though he said he mashed and fermented out most of the barley flavor.

Given the requisite addition of barley malt to Chateau Jiahu, Dogfish Head's concoction is classified as a beer, Calagione said. However, McGovern said the beverage made in China 9,000 years ago defies description. "We called it a mixed beverage, because we're not sure where it fits in," he said.

Gerhart too struggled to categorize the beverage. "It wasn't a beer, but it was, it wasn't a mead, yet it was and it sure wasn't a wine or a cider. It was somewhere between all of them, in this gray area," he said.

Visually, Gerhart described Chateau Jiahu as gold in color with a dense, white head similar to champagne bubbles. Calagione said the beverage most closely resembles a Belgian-style ale.

According to McGovern, the brew is "very intriguing" with a taste and aroma of the grape and hawthorn fruits. To better match the 9,000-year-old beverage, however, he said it should probably be sweeter. "Sugar is relatively rare in nature, yet we're very much attracted to it. We're also attracted to alcohol—all animals are attracted to these substances. The ancient Chinese would have wanted to retain as much sugar as they could. They would have had a sweet tooth," he said.

Dogfish Head sold out its first batch of Chateau Jiahu. Most was consumed at a May debut dinner at the Waldorf-Astoria hotel in New York City, the remainder quickly drunk at the Milton brewery by beer fans of exotic beer.

Calagione hopes to brew up a larger batch this fall and, potentially, to market it widely, as he has Midas Touch.

Beer in Ancient Mesopotamia

While no one can be exactly sure how the process of beer making was discovered or who first discovered it, most historians think that some bread or grain was left unattended and somehow got wet, fermenting into an inebriating pile of mush thanks to yeast in the air. One has to wonder at the thought process of the person tasting the result for the first time, perhaps it was a dare between fun-loving Mesopotamian frat boys... or more likely it was simply that up until very recently, no one would have dreamed of wasting any food, even a pile of putrid mush. If there was a way to make it palatable and it didn't kill you, people would use it to avoid waste.

Beer has a long history, one that's longer than we'll ever be able to trace. Residue of the first known barley beer was found in a jar at the Godin Tepe excavation site in modern day Iran, presumably sitting there since some ancient Sumerian took his or her last sip around 3400 BC. But chances are, the first beer "formula" had been "cracked" millennia before that.

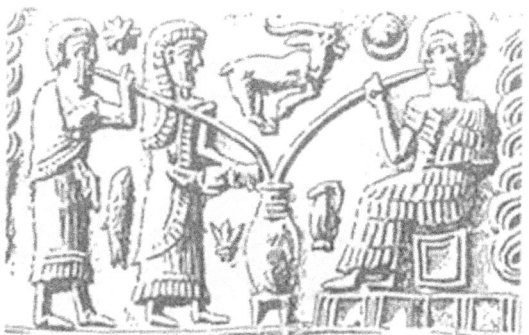

So, while an exact date or time for the first chug, or keg stand, or even hiccup, is not known, what *is* known is that beer, like bread, developed best in farm-based, agrarian societies where there was an enough grain and time for fermentation. One thing we *definitely* know is that ancient

Ancient Babylonians drinking beer through straws

man loved beer as much as—if not more—than we do: the Babylonians had about 20 recipes for beer.

As almost any substance containing certain sugars can undergo spontaneous fermentation due to wild yeasts in the air, it is probable that beer-like beverages were independently invented nearly at the same time among various cultures throughout the world. Chemical tests of ancient pottery jars reveal that beer was already being produced about 7,000 years ago in China and what is today Iran.

In Mesopotamia, the oldest evidence of beer is believed to be a 6,000-year-old Sumerian tablet depicting people drinking a beverage through reed straws from a communal bowl. A 3900-year-old Sumerian poem honoring Ninkasi, the patron goddess of brewing, contains the oldest surviving beer recipe, describing the production of beer from barley via bread.

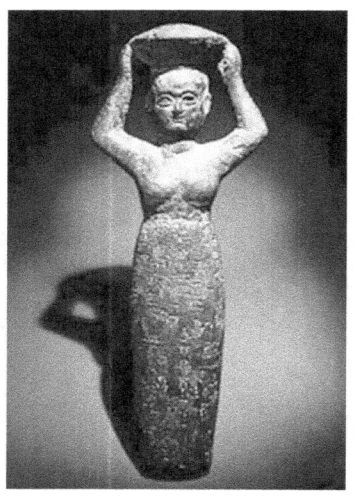

Ninkasi, you are the one who bakes the bappir in the big oven, Puts in order the piles of hulled grains.

You are the one who waters the malt set on the ground...
You are the one who holds with both hands the great sweet wort...

Ninkasi, you are the one who pours out the filtered beer of the collector vat, It is [like] the onrush of Tigris and Euphrates.

The people of ancient Mesopotamia enjoyed beer so much that it was a daily dietary staple. Paintings, poems, and myths depict both human beings and their gods enjoying beer which was consumed through a straw to filter out pieces of bread or herbs in the drink. The brew was thick, of the consistency of modern-day porridge, and the straw was invented by the Sumerians or the Babylonians, it is thought, specifically for the purpose of drinking beer. The famous poem *Inanna and the God of Wisdom* describes the two deities drinking beer together and the god of wisdom, Enki, becoming so drunk he gives away the sacred *meh* (laws of civilization) to Inanna (thought to symbolize the transfer of power from Eridu, the city of Enki, to Uruk, the city of Inanna).

The Sumerian poem *Hymn to Ninkasi*, above, is both a song of praise to the goddess of beer, Ninkasi, and a recipe for beer, first written down around 1800 BC. In the Sumerian/Babylonian *Epic of Gilgamesh*, the hero Enkidu becomes civilized through the efforts and ministrations of the temple harlot Shamhat who, among other things, teaches him to drink beer.

The Sumerians had many different words for beer from `sikaru' to `dida' to `ebir' (which meant `beer mug') and regarded the drink as a gift from the gods to promote human happiness and well-being. The original brewers were women, the priestesses of Ninkasi, and women brewed beer regularly in the home as part of their preparation of meals. Beer was made from bippar (twice-baked barley bread) which was then fermented and beer brewing was always associated with baking. The famous Alulu beer receipt from the city of Ur in 2050 BC, however, shows that beer brewing had become commercialized by that time. The tablet acknowledges receipt of 5 Silas of `the best beer' from the brewer Alulu (five Silas being approximately four and a half litres).

The temples issued workers with daily rations of barley beer, the

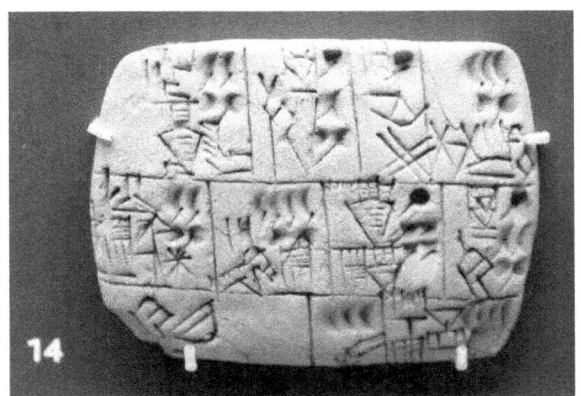

staple drink of Mesopotamia. The tablet on the left was impressed with five different types of numerical symbol. From Mesopotamia, Iraq. Late Uruk Period, 3100-3000 BC. (Photo courtesy of The British Museum, London)

21

Under Babylonian rule, Mesopotamian beer production increased dramatically, became more commercialized, and laws were instituted concerning it as paragraphs 108-110 of the Code of Hammurabi make clear:

108

If a tavern-keeper (feminine) does not accept corn according to gross weight in payment of drink, but takes money, and the price of the drink is less than that of the corn, she shall be convicted and thrown into the water.

109

If conspirators meet in the house of a tavern-keeper, and these conspirators are not captured and delivered to the court, the tavern-keeper shall be put to death.

110

If a "sister of a god" open a tavern, or enter a tavern to drink, then shall this woman be burned to death.

Law 108 had to do with those tavern keepers who poured `short measures' of beer in return for cash instead of corn (which could be weighed and held to a measure) to cheat their customers; they would be drowned if caught doing so. Beer was commonly used in barter, not for cash sale and a daily ration of beer was provided for all citizens, the amount depending on one's social status. The second law concerns tavern keepers encouraging treason by allowing malcontents to gather in their establishment and the third law cited concerns women who were consecrated to, or were priestesses of, a certain deity opening a common drinking house or drinking in an already established tavern. The Babylonians had nothing against a priestess drinking beer (as, with the Sumerians, beer was considered a gift from the gods) but objected to one doing so in the same way as common women would.

The Babylonians brewed many different kinds of beer and classified them into twenty categories which recorded their various characteristics. Beer became a regular commodity in foreign trade, especially with Egypt, where it was very popular.

Beer in Ancient Egypt

We know that the ancient Egyptians enjoyed the benefits of beer, Egyptian Pharaohs were buried with vats of the stuff, even the workers who built the pyramids were essentially *paid* in beer. An authentic ancient Egyptian beer, which we today call Tutankhamun Ale, was replicated and brewed from emmer wheat by the Courage Brewery in 1996.

The Egyptian goddess of beer was Tenenit (closely associated with Meskhenet, goddess of childbirth and protector of the birthing house) whose name derives from *tenemu*, one of the Egyptian words for beer. The most popular beer in Egypt was *Heqet* (or *Hecht*) which was a honey-flavored brew and their word for beer in general was *zytum*. The workers at the Giza plateau received beer rations three times a day and beer was often used throughout Egypt as compensation for labor. The Egyptians believed that brewing was taught to human beings by the great god Osiris himself and in this, and other regards, they viewed beer in much the same way as the Mesopotamians did. As in Mesopotamia, women were the chief brewers at first and brewed in their homes, the beer initially had the same thick, porridge-like consistency, and was brewed in much the same way. Later, men took over the business of brewing and miniature carved figures found in the tomb of Meketre (Prime Minister to the pharaoh Mentuhotep II, 2050-2000 BCE) show an ancient brewery at work (see below).

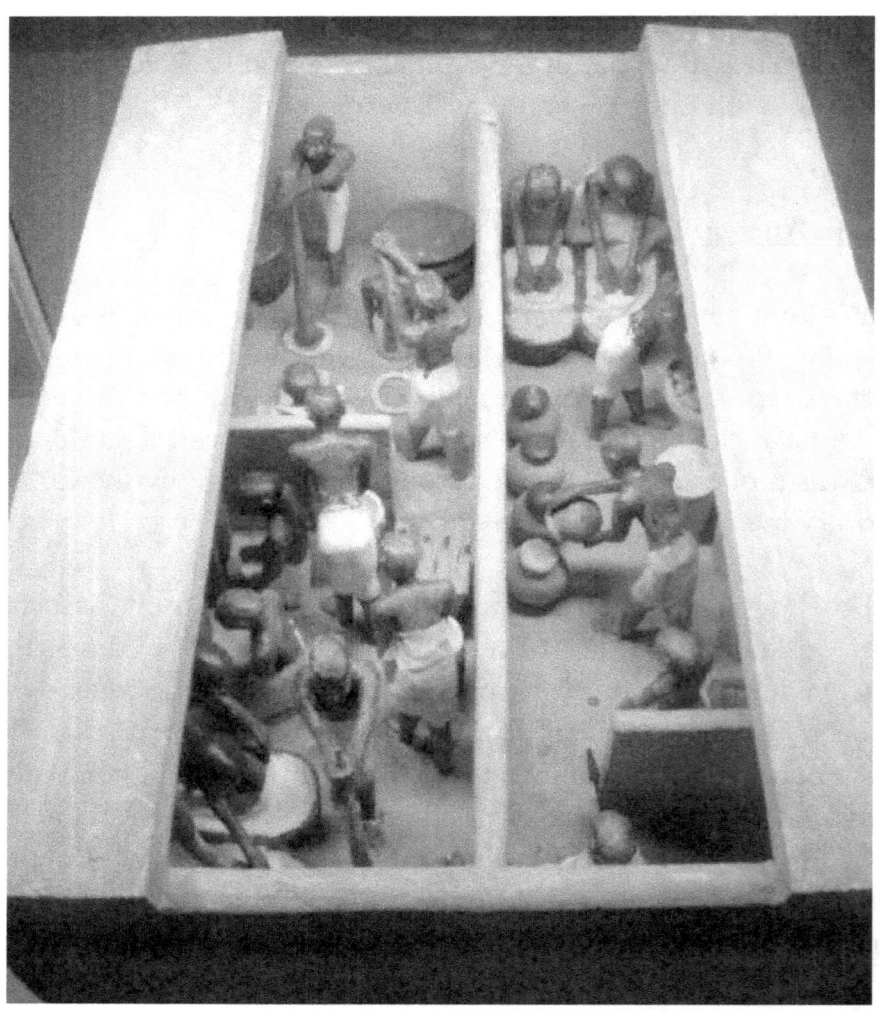

According to the Metropolitan Museum of Art, describing the diorama, "The overseer with a baton sits inside the door. In the brewery two women grind flour, which another man works into dough. After a second man treads the dough into mash in a tall vat, it is put into tall crocks to ferment. After fermentation, it is poured off into round jugs with black clay stoppers."

Beer played an integral role in the very popular myth of the birth of the goddess Hathor. According to the tale (which has much in it which pre-dates the biblical tale of the Great Flood in Genesis) the god Ra, incensed at the evil and ingratitude of humanity, sends Sekhmet to earth to destroy his creation. He repents of his decision, however, as Sekhmet's blood lust grows with the destruction of every town and city. He has a great quantity of beer dyed red and dropped at the city of Dendera where Sekhmet, thinking it is a huge pool of blood, stops her rampage to drink. She gets drunk, falls asleep, and wakes as the goddess Hathor, the benevolent deity of, among other things, music, laughter, the sky and, especially, gratitude. The association between gratitude, Hathor and beer, is highlighted by an inscription from 2200 BCE found at Dendera, Hathor's cult center: "The mouth of a perfectly contented man is filled with beer." Beer was enjoyed so regularly among the Egyptians that Queen Cleopatra VII lost popularity toward the end of her reign more for implementing a tax on beer (the first ever) than for her wars with Rome which the beer tax went to help pay for (although she claimed the tax was to deter public drunkeness). As beer was often prescribed for medicinal purposes (there were over 100 remedies using beer) the tax was considered unjust.

Beer is also mentioned in the Epic of Gilgamesh. Beer became vital to all the grain-growing civilizations of classical Western antiquity, including Egypt — so much so that in 1868 James Death put forward a theory in '*The Beer of the Bible*' that the manna from heaven that God gave the Israelites was a bread-based, porridge-like beer called wusa. The modern anthropologist Alan Eames believes that "beer was the driving force that led nomadic mankind into village life...It was this appetite for beer-making material that led to crop cultivation, permanent settlement and agriculture."

I don't know about all of that but I do know that knowledge of brewing was passed on to the Greeks. Plato wrote that "He was a wise man who invented beer." The Greeks then taught the Romans to brew. The Romans called their brew "*cerevisia*," from Ceres, the goddess of agriculture, and *vis*, Latin for "strength."

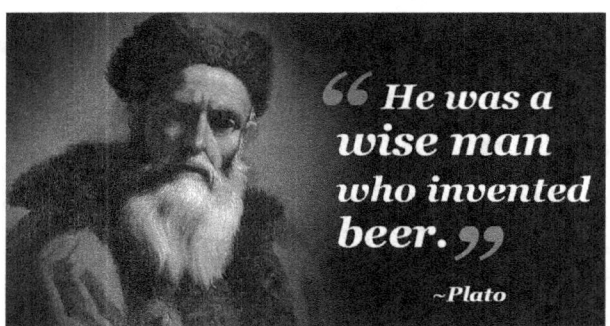

Beer was important to early Romans, but during Republican times wine displaced beer as the preferred alcoholic beverage. Beer became a beverage considered fit only for barbarians; Tacitus wrote disparagingly of the beer brewed by the Germanic peoples of his day. Calling it, "…a weak and inferior liquid produced by a weak and inferior people."

Thracians were also known to consume beer made from rye, even since the 5th century BC, as Hellanicus of Lesbos says in operas. Their name for beer was brutos, or brytos. In short, various types and brews of beer have been imbibed by every recorded civilization of mankind but none more than one particular people… The Germans.

But perhaps I am jumping ahead of things here. Any discussion of beer must begin with the two simple understandings, one, is that the history of beer necessitates a look at the history of all that is

German and two, that Beer—any beer—is a truly simple beverage. All you need is some malted grain, a good dose of water, a smidgen of flavorings, a bit of yeast, and, voila, you've got beer. It is the brewer's art, and a true art it is, that turns these simple materials into a sheer endless variety of divine gustatory pleasures.

Beverages, like food, are always symbols of the culinary culture in which they emerged. The greatest drinks are pearls of civilization that have matured over centuries. When we think of Champagne, Cabernet Sauvignon or Cognac, for instance, we conjure up images of the 'joie de vie' of the French. When we savor a Sherry or a Malaga, we are partaking in the mystery that is southern Spain. How could a frozen Vodka be 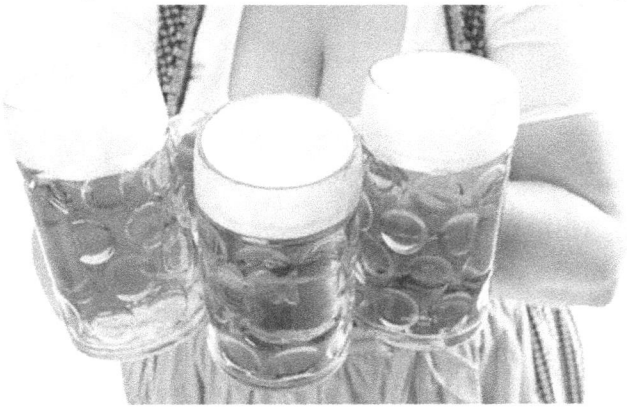 anything but Russian or a Tequila anything but Mexican? Likewise, when we drink a Munich Helles or an Oktoberfestbier, we are vicariously transported into the lederhosen-slapping land of the Bavarians. The character of the drink seems always a reflection of the character of the people who created it.

It may come as a surprise to modern beer enthusiasts, to learn that the history of German beer has been, for the most part, one of ale, not lager -- in spite of the present-day preponderance of blond lagers, which currently hold well over two-thirds of the German beer market. But if you scratch the surface of the German lager veneer, what you'll find is a bed rock of solid ale traditions. Until the 16th century all German beer was ale. Until about the eighth century, it was brewed almost exclusively in the home, by tribal hausfraus, yes, it is thanks to women that we have beer! By the 11th century it was brewed mostly by professional brew monks and brew nuns, until feudal lords took over most institutional brewing in southern Germany, while burgher-merchants did the same in northern Germany.

Germans have been brewing ales for at least three thousand years, but lagers (specifically: brown lagers) for only five centuries. The blond, crisp, clean lagers, for which Germans have become so famous in our age, have been around for a scant 150 years. The now ubiquitous hoppy Pils started its conquest only about 30 years ago.

Thus, do not judge history by the most recent past, lest you take as fact what might be a fad or a short-term trend. Decades, even centuries, do not mean all that much in a country, where a traveler can eat and drink in places that were already old when Columbus sailed the seas and discovered that there was an entire continent blocking his route to the orient. There are pubs in Germany, where centuries of stolid bums have rubbed cozy, indelible hollows into wooden benches, from which a contemporary imbiber can take unobtrusive support and comfort as he settles in for an evening of delectable degustation. *Dégustation*, by the way, is a culinary term meaning a careful, appreciative tasting of various foods and focusing on the gustatory system, the senses, high culinary art and good company... (Don't I sound smug! Don't be fooled – I had to look up the term too!)

In Germany, the fortunes of beer have always been intimately intertwined with the ups and downs of the country's political and religious history, but the secular and the sacred have been strange bed fellows, each with the capacity to reach down into the everyday life of common man and to regulate his existence from cradle to grave.

The secular authorities build roads, collect taxes, train armies, mete out justice, mint coins, finance welfare and organize the police, while the churches preach morals, baptize babies, bury the dead, set up schools and hospitals and give to the poor. But at certain times in history, religious leaders, in competition with their secular counterparts, also had their own armies, sources of tax revenue, courts of law, territorial claims and commercial enterprises. What does this have to do with German beer, you may ask? The answer is: everything! In a culture where beer defines part of the national character, the question of who controls the brew is paramount. He who has his hand on the levers of power, also has his thumb in the people's beer mug.

One can trace the roots of German beer making back to the tribal Germanic marauders of yore. These inhabitants of the dark Teutonic forests used to menace the poor Roman legionnaires who were sent there to do Caesar's bidding. As we know from Roman reports, Germanic hausfrau-brewsters minded the kettle in the forest clearings. Yes, home brewing had been a venerable tradition on this earth long before February 1979, when Jimmy Carter repealed its prohibition in the United States.

Between the 6th and the 9th centuries, the tribal societies of central Europe became both Christianized and organized into countries united by language and customs. This set the stage for a

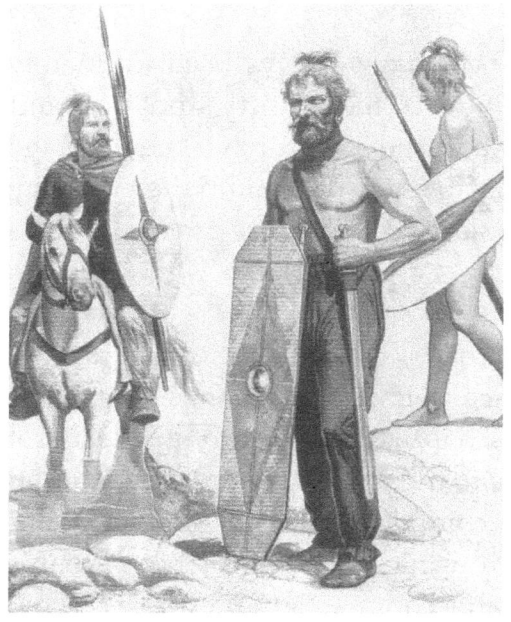

power struggle between the secular feudal lords and the Christian bishops and monks for control over all facets of life--including beer making! By the 11th century, monastic breweries, run mostly by Benedictine monks and nuns, enjoyed an almost exclusive right to brew and sell beer.

By the 12th century, the feudals, possessed by greed and envy and always strapped for revenues, began to take back most of the brew privileges they had granted so generously to the religious orders during the previous centuries. Many a lord started his own Hofbräuhaus (or court brew house). While the struggle between the feudals and the clerics over the spoils of power was at its most ferocious, both parties seemed to have missed the rise, at the beginning of the second millennium, of a new, third force in society, which was ultimately to snatch the economic prize out of both their clutches.

This emerging new force were the enterprising city burghers, who quietly created a new prosperity based on industry, commerce and technological innovation. Within a few centuries, they had all but monopolized the making of top quality beers with great taste and keeping qualities. They erected private trading empires that spanned most of the known world of the time, and beer, next to minerals, furs and dry goods was among their most profitable commodities. Through their ventures, these free-spirited burghers planted the seeds of our modern civilization that would, in due course, limit the clergy to its spiritual purpose and relegate the nobles to the historical junk heap.

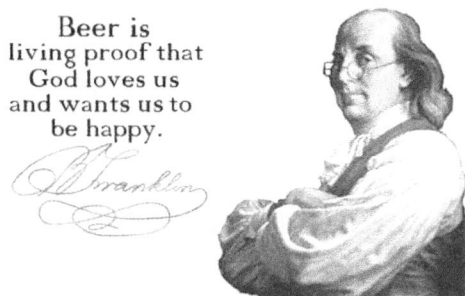

Beer is living proof that God loves us and wants us to be happy.

Franklin

The development of German beer as we know it today was virtually finished by the time the 20th century rolled around, as were the struggles for political and economic power between church and state and between the common people and the aristocrats. But for about a thousand years, the question of who ran the country and owned the beer; monks, lords, merchants, or guilds, had determined which beers were brewed and distributed, and in which quantity and of which quality. Church, state and free enterprise each had its fair share in either furthering or retarding the progress of German beer. From (literally) murky beginnings at the dawn of European civilization, German beers have evolved into mature, sophisticated brews with an unmistakable character that stems from a unique combination of ingredients and processes.

Let me take you on a journey of discovery so that next time you pop open a bottle of German beer, you can savor not only its sublime complexity, but also the story behind it. Come with me now as we journey to the dawn of German Beer. If you want to skip this rather lengthy history of beer in Germany jump ahead to page 119 to continue with a brief history of beer in the United States or to page 134 to look into the health benefits that chocolate, wine, and beer have to offer us!

2 Beer in Germany

A 'Not so Brief' German Beer History

The tribal inhabitants of northern and central Europe started to make beer from wheat, barley or any other grain that grew wild and was considered of not much use for anything else, as early as the latter part of the Bronze Age, probably before 1000 B.C. This we know from their sagas and myths. At that time, Celtic and Germanic tribes were competing for control over patches of inhabitable space in the forests. The struggle between the two groups lasted until about the fourth century BC, when the Germans had either ousted the Celts from the continent or had assimilated them. Only on the British Isles and along the Atlantic coast of present-day France did the Celts remain the dominant cultural force for another millennium or so.

The tribes of central Europe, spread out over such a large territory and with very little communication among them, naturally were less homogeneous than the collective term "German" implies. The Danes, Norwegians and Swedes of Scandinavia evolved their distinct "Norse" culture, while the inhabitants of Caesar's gallia (roughly modern France and Belgium) developed their "Gallic" ways. Only the tribes in the very center; prominent among them the Alemans, Swabians, Bavarians and Saxons, created a culture that we now associate with the term "German." But no matter where the Germans lived and what their customs, they were brewers all!

The pagans of northern Europe called their beer öl, which is the root of the modern word "ale". But since these folks could neither read nor write, we have no firm documentary evidence of the beginnings of their ale. We do know for sure, however, that the Germans were already regular ale brewers by about 800 B.C. Archaeologists have uncovered the burial site of a well-to-do German of that time, near the Franconian village of Kasendorf, seven miles from Kulmbach, in northern Bavaria. The grave not only contained the remains of the deceased gentleman but also the provisions his contemporaries had generously supplied for his trip into the realm of the spirits. Among these were crocks of beer, which, when unearthed almost 3,000 years later, still contained traces of bread, the standard raw material for the mashes of ancient times.

Today, Kulmbach is home to many famous brews, including the Kulmbacher Mönchshof Kloster Schwarzbier, a malty black lager. Founded as a monastery brewery in 1349 and secularized in 1791, the Mönchshof brewery is still going strong as part of the Kulmbacher Reichelbräu conglomerate. Surely, almost 3,000 years of virtually uninterrupted brewing in the Kulmbach region must constitute a world record!

Early beers were usually dark brews "mashed" from half-baked loaves of bread made from coarsely-ground barley or wheat. The gentle, moist baking of the loaves probably had a similar effect on the grain as today's malting, that is, of activating the enzymes required for the conversion of starches into fermentable sugars. This "modified" bread was then soaked in crocks filled with water, where it fermented. The result was a murky and sour ale, full of floating husks and crumbs--a far cry from the clean and crisp beers made in Germany today. The first truly historical accounts of beer making among the Germans came from their Roman conquerors—those literate, wine-drinking military men and imperial officials, who reveled in exposing the deplorable predilection of the barbarian germanii for their inferior "barley wines." These, by Roman standards, were second-rate beverages, often flavored with such unspeakables as oak bark, aspen leaves or even the content of an oxen's gall bladder.

At the time of the first Roman contact, the Germans were already producing beer in large quantities. Thus, the Greco-Roman geographer Strabo (around 63 B.C. - 21 A.D.) wrote, when he reported that one tribe, the Cimbri, used bronze brew kettles capable of holding about 500 liters. Today, we would call this a 4¼-barrel brewhouse. "A remarkable metallurgical achievement for that time!"

Some historians speculate that Julius Caesar and his legions learned about beer making from the Germans and introduced it to the British Isles in 55 or 53 BC, but other historians insist that the Celts had mastered the art of ale making on their own, long before the Romans had figured out how to cross the British Channel in boats. Suffice it to say that, around the birth of Christ, ale was the most popular drink of all the Europeans north of the Alps.

The best description of tribal Germanic drinking habits has come to us from the Roman historian Publius Cornelius Tacitus. In his '_De origine et situ germanorum_' (About the origin and location of the Germans), which he completed in 98 A.D., Tacitus asserted, with some contempt, that the Germanic folk were proficient imbibers, who sought out even the slightest excuse for 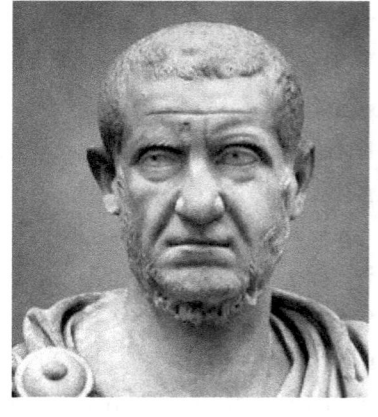 having a drinking party. No other people, he wrote, were inclined to enjoy so much the art of banqueting and entertaining as the

Germans, and it was customary for them to invite strangers into their homes to share a meal and a brew. "The germanii," he said, "serve an extract of barley and rye as a beverage that is somehow adulterated (presumably he means: fermented) to resemble wine."

Perhaps, the cartoon cliché of raucous tribesmen, frolicking on their bear skins in front of a camp fire and passing, from one eager mouth to the next, their richly ornamented aurochs horns filled with intoxicating liquids, is not too far-fetched after all. Tacitus was impressed by the vigor and energy of the Germans. He described the country as rough and crude, the air as unpleasant, but the people, although inferior to the Romans, he considered to be pure and unspoiled. He observed that the men were capable of withstanding cold and hunger and were always ready to attempt feats of daring. There was one deprivation, however, the Germans apparently could not bear: THIRST! No wonder that both honey beer (mead) and grain beer always flowed in copious quantities at important tribal gatherings, where the Germans discussed such weighty matters as war and peace or the betrothal of a chieftain's daughter.

The Germans sure knew how to have fun and, contrary to current perceptions of their 20th century descendants, were none too eager to do heavy work. At least this is what Tacitus wanted us to believe. He even suggested that it might have been easier to conquer the germanii by shipments of cerevisia (beer) than by force of pilum (lance) and gladius (sword):

"If we wanted to make use of their addiction to drink, by giving them as much of it as they want, we could defeat them as easily by means of this vice as with our weapons...They cultivate the grains of the field with much greater patience and perseverance than one would expect from them, in light of their customary laziness."

In Roman high society, German beer was held in such disdain that even the Emperor Flavius Claudius Julianus (331 - 363 AD) felt himself called upon to rhyme a silly ditty about the superior virtues of wine compared to beer. In his poem, he likened the smell of wine to that of nectar and the smell of the Germanic "drink from grain" to that of a billy goat. Julianus had come to know the Germans and their beer from his many battles against the Franks and Alemans. Unimpressed by the highbrow Roman attitude, however, the tribal marauders of the Gallic and Teutonic forests continued to down their indigenous beverages just as they continued to menace the poor legionnaires sent from the Apennine peninsula to keep an eye on them. The sylvan primitives proved to be intrepid warriors, who were as fond of draining the life blood out of their sophisticated, wine-drinking oppressors as they were of draining their aurochs horns of murky quaff. For the emissaries of mighty Rome, life was never safe at such camps as colonia claudia ara agrippinensium (today's Cologne), castra novesia (today's Neuß, outside Düsseldorf), castra xantippa (today's Xanten, on the Rhine, near the Dutch border) or treveris (today's Trier at the Moselle River, near Luxembourg).

The Romans had brought the grape to central Europe so that they could indulge in the drinking habits to which they were accustomed at home. But it is obvious that eventually they developed a taste for the "inferior" beverage of their Germanic underlings. How else are we to interpret the tomb stone of a Roman merchant, who died in treveris (Trier) on the Moselle River, in 260 A.D.? The epitaph on his stone identifies him as a cervesarius, a beer merchant. Founded by Emperor Augustus in 15 BC, treveris was the capital of the western part of the Roman Empire and served as administrative headquarters of the Roman territories from Spain to Britain. In this great city of the world, our cervesarius had his liquid wares privately brewed by German ladies in the neighborhood and sold the merchandise at a fine mark-up to his civilized Roman customers.

The Romans even learned to brew themselves, as is evident from a complete Roman brewery discovered in 1983 near the Bavarian city of Regensburg, on the banks of the Danube. This brewery dates from the 2nd or 3rd century A.D. and was part of a canaba, a settlement of craftsmen, that had sprung up within the walls of a fortification called castra regina (hence the modern name of the city: Regensburg). Castra regina was built in 179 A.D. by the Roman Emperor Marcus Aurelius. Because of its strategic location along the north-eastern flank of the empire, it became the largest Roman camp in what is now southern Germany, housing some 6,000, obviously thirsty, legionnaires as well as scores of administrators and support personnel.

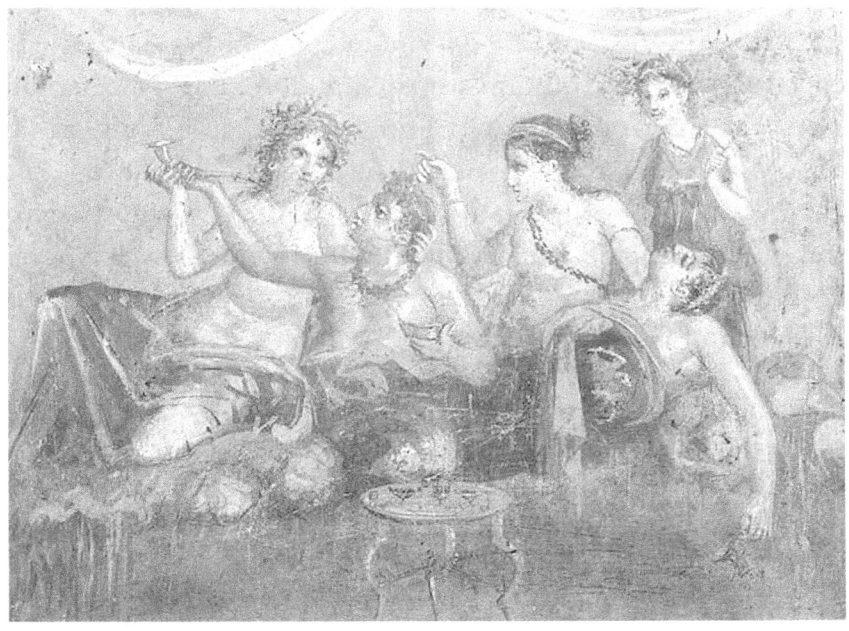

It is apparent from the construction of the kiln and mash tun of the Regensburg brewery that German beer making had, by that time, progressed from the primitive bread beer found in the grave near Kulmbach to the mashing of malted grains as we practice it today.

Evidence of another Roman brewery in Germany, a fermenter with residues of black beer, was found in 1911 during the excavation of a Roman camp near Alzey, in Germany's largest wine-growing region, in the state of Rhineland-Palatine. Apparently, the fermenter and its contents were hastily abandoned by the Romans sometime in the year in 353 AD, during a surprise attack by the Alemans.

The Romans' ultimate embrace of the barbaric beverage is also reflected in their language. They came to regard beer as a gift from Ceres, the goddess of agriculture, and treasured it as a strength-giving potion (vis = strength). Hence their term for beer: cerevisia.

We are now peeking into the sixth century AD. The Roman Empire had crumbled and the Germanic way of life had flourished in the clearings of the Teutonic forest and along the river banks. For the next three centuries, life, when not interrupted by raiding Huns, Vikings or Saracens, would generally be peaceful in the little farming villages up and down the lands of the Franks, Alemans, Saxons, Swabians, Thuringians and Bavarians. Indigenous civilizations, no longer under the yoke of Latin legions and their own version of pax romana, began to take shape.

While the man of the house was out tending his fields of barley and wheat or chasing the stag in the woods, the lady of the house was busy at the domestic hearth making the bread, the stew and the brew. In German families of that period, home brewing was as ubiquitous as home cooking and baking, and the brew kettle was as important a part of a maiden's dowry as were her cooking pots and pans. It was customary for a brewster-hausfrau to invite her neighbors to a round of afternoon beer. The ladies took the beverage with pieces of bread dunked into it, perhaps a forerunner of the modern coffee-klatsch?

This was the epoch when two influences of tremendous impact on the fate of German brewing began to emerge: feudalism and Christianity. Feudalism established controls from above that changed brewing in Germany from a household activity of the common folk into a privileged commercial activity of a favored few, practiced first mostly by monks and nuns and, since the 12th century, more and more by secular court breweries and mercantile enterprises.

The other influence, Christianity, brought with it the emergence of monasteries not only as beneficiaries of the privileges doled out by the secular lords, but also as centers of education and learning, where brewing knowledge could accumulate, quality standards could improve, and the craft of brewing could evolve, for the first time in Europe, into a true profession.

Effective power in the Dark Ages resided in local dukes, appointed by the king and pledged to him by a personal oath of fealty. These vassals were charged with raising armies for defense and public safety and carrying out administrative and judicial duties. In exchange, the local lords received land, which they, in turn, subdivided into smaller holdings run by subvassals and worked by serfs. The vassals owed their immediate overlords obedience, war service and a prescribed number of soldiers, usually recruited from the ranks of the serfs. The bold and strong eventually rose to become noble knights and the weak sank to become toiling peasants. In time, social positions became hereditary and the system evolved into pure feudalism, a static, money-less form of exchange, in which the folks at the bottom traded their labor and their freedom for security and protection provided by those at the top.

Such was the system that Charlemagne found, when he started his reign in 768 AD. With few means of transportation and communication, an emperor rarely stayed put for long in the capital, which was Aachen (or Aix-la-Chapelle), about 40 miles west of Cologne. Rulers looked after the realm and local matters by traveling from one castle or crown estate to the next. Without much money in circulation, taxes were in the form of the fruits of the land. The emperor traveled to his revenues in order to consume them on location, since he could not have them travel to him in the form of coins for his treasury.

Charlemagne's empire was organized into great estates, each with a master's house, church, grain mill, forge, bakery, stables, barns, workshops, peasant's cottages and, of course, a brewery. Charlemagne was a great supporter of 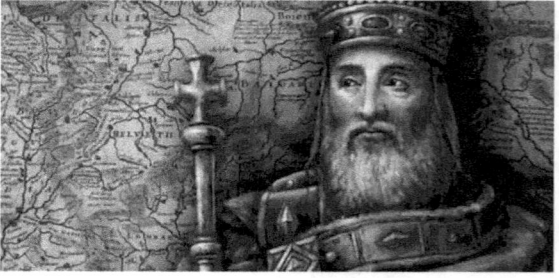 the brewing craft and insisted that there be a brewery in each of his estates. For his vassals, he wrote an elaborate set of economic ordinances, entitled 'Capitulare caroli magni de villis' (The main points about running Charlemagne's estates), in which he gave rather detailed instructions about almost any aspect of management, including that of the brewery.

Whenever he showed up, paragraph 61 kicked in:
"We wish that the intendant on duty bring before Our Person samples of beer. We also wish that they bring along their brew

master so that they can brew for Us good beer in our presence."

In paragraph 34, he instructed brewers about hygiene:
"The administrators have to make sure that workers who use their hands in the preparation of beer, keep themselves especially clean."

He also insisted on annual reports (paragraph 62):
"We also wish that our intendants compose an annual inventory ledger at Christmas time. We also want a list of the beers they brew so that we know which quantities of the different products are available."

In these ordinances lie the seeds of institutional, commercial brewing in central Europe, an activity in which the monasteries were soon to become the most successful players.

At the time of Charlemagne, monasteries were a recent innovation. Outside Italy, the first people to be Christianized were the Irish and the Britons, early in the fifth century. Imbued with missionary zeal, the new converts set out to save continental pagans from damnation. By the beginning of the sixth century, Irish missionaries had started to penetrate the heathen Teutonic forests in search of souls. They founded small monasteries from which they spread the gospel. A particularly successful missionary was the Irish Saint Columban, who, with his band of followers, planted the seeds of the new creed in parts of present-day France, Austria, Germany and Switzerland. At St. Gall, in Switzerland, a disciple of his founded the famous monastery that was to become by far the largest brewery of the Dark Ages. Another famous missionary/brewer was the Franconian monk Corbinian, who, in 724, built a simple chapel on Weihenstephan Mountain, north of Munich. He must have picked a great spot, since the little religious outpost grew into a Benedictine Abbey, which, in 1040, obtained, from Bishop Engilbert of Freising, official brewing privileges and the right to sell its beer for profit. Today, the brewery at Weihenstephan is owned by the State of Bavaria and is the oldest continuously operating brewery in the world.

Like all Germanic households, the good brethren of the early Middle Ages grew their own grain and made their own brew. They soon discovered that beer, if made strong enough and from the best grains, was not only thirst quenching but also very nourishing, a veritable "liquid bread." This was important to the monks because of their penchant for periodic fasting, when no solid food was permitted to pass their lips. Liquids, however, did not break the fast, at least according to ecclesiastic doctrine, which was made up by the church fathers in Rome. The Holy See, of course, knew little about German beer. Nunneries, too, became centers of institutional brewing. After all, their inhabitants would have become secular beer-making hausfraus had they not chosen the nun's habit.

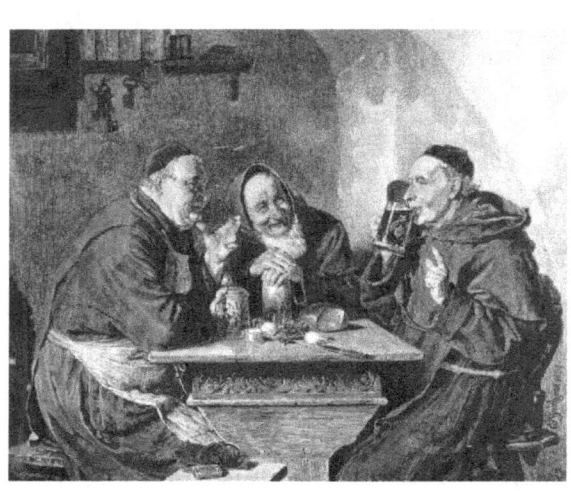

The monks and nuns made more beer than they needed just for their own consumption. As part of their charitable works, they shared both their bread and their beer with the poor and with any traveler or pilgrim who might ask for shelter. Soon, monastery beer gained a reputation for quality. As the demand increased, so did the size of the monastic breweries, and some brothers and sisters began to specialize in brewery work.

Being well-educated people, the friars and nuns took a scientific approach to brewing. They experimented with new techniques and ingredients and created systematic records of the results. In the process, they discovered the virtues of hops as a bittering and preserving agent, though nobody is quite sure exactly when, and probably developed the first beers of consistently high quality. We know that, already in the eighth century, the monastery of Weihenstephan was surrounded by hop gardens, and it is doubtful that the friars cultivated the vine merely for aesthetic reasons.

In a book entitled 'Physica sacra' (Sacred world), we can find the first written description of the preserving and healthful effects of hops in beer. The book's author is Hildegard von Bingen (1098 - 1179), a Benedictine abbess, brew nun, physician, natural scientist, and advisor to Emperor Frederick I (a.k.a. Barbarossa). Hildegard drank beer regularly and lived to be 81 years old, an incredible age for that time. It is not surprising that some people like to see a causal connection between her longevity and her dedication to beer.

From kings to serfs, the inhabitants of the feudal world eventually grew to fear the material and spiritual weapons of the church. Otto strengthened the church's position by granting it feudal lay rights and privileges, including the gruit right. Soon, the monastic brewers of the early Middle Ages began to enjoy connections in high places. We know that in 947, for instance, Otto I himself conferred the gruit right upon the church of Liége (in present-day Belgium). Higher-up ecclesiastics became themselves grantors of the gruit right to their subordinates, as did the Bishop of Metz (in present-day France), when he conferred the gruit right onto the nearby monastery of St. Trond, and the Bishop of Cologne, when he gave it to the church of Neuß (near the present-day Alt beer home of Düsseldorf).

After the demise of Rome, it fell upon the Christian monks to hold the Western world together. Sheltered behind their monastery walls, the friars created little paradises, refuges in the wilderness, where they copied old books, wrote new ones, conducted almost the only schools and, generally, preserved culture and learning during the five centuries of economic and cultural stagnation that we call the Dark Ages.

Like the feudal manors around them, medieval monasteries were virtually self-sufficient. They grew their own grain, raised their own meat, baked their own bread, brewed their own beer. They lived and worked simply, believing that meals should be simple and never large. Food and drink should sustain life, not harm it. **Drunkenness was forbidden** and the monk who spilled beer had to stand upright and still for an entire night.

Trade in the Dark Ages was mostly carried out by itinerant peddlers who visited settlements on foot or with pack animals. But they had much to contend with: horrible roads, inclement elements, thievish landlords, piracy, and brigands. The monasteries were often the safest refuge for a weary traveler. With Christian fervor on the upswing, pilgrimages, too, became very popular, with Rome and Jerusalem claiming the top of the charts for holy destinations. The hooded fishermen of souls, with hostels and breweries already in place along the old Roman roads, went into the hospitality business with gusto.

As the flow of pilgrims and other traveling folk increased on the highways and byways of the empire, so did the monasteries' operations. The food, drink and shelter the monks used to share out of charity with anyone who came, soon became a commodity offered to the dusty travelers for profit. Not surprisingly, the observance of ascetic rules began to take a back seat to the chores of providing for the itinerant customers. After a day of hard work in the monasteries' fields, kitchens and 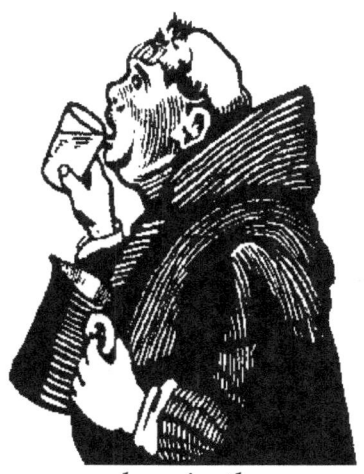 breweries, many a monk naturally found more solace in the merry company of his guests than in the austere cloister regimen prescribed by that seemingly so un-Irish Irishman St. Columban.

Shielded by feudal rights and privileges and confronted with an ever-increasing demand for their brews, many an abbot eventually succumbed to the commercial temptation and started to sell beer for profit. Cloister inns and pubs began to do a roaring business. Every monastery brewed a different beer and tried to corner the market. The spiritual comrade in the good lord's army soon became the commercial competitor in the beverage business down the road.

Economically, monastic breweries were much like secular businesses, but with several competitive advantages: cheap or free raw materials, cheap or free labor and exemption from all taxes. Monastery beer was good and it was cheap. No wonder that some of these breweries became truly gigantic. The cloister inn at Nürnberg, it is chronicled, eventually made as much as 4,500 buckets (about 2,500 barrels) of beer per year! Another in Bavaria served close to 10,000 guests a year.

The 10th and 11th centuries were the heyday of monastic brewing in Germany. In a country of perhaps nine or ten million inhabitants, there were some 500 monastery breweries (300 of which were located in Bavaria alone) producing beer in unsurpassed quantity and quality. And all the beer was ale. The commercialization of the monastic brew not only propelled it to high standards, but also lead to its eventual downfall. Ultimately, the monasteries became victims of the envy and opposition that their own successes had bred. The riches garnered from the brewing trade enabled the cloistered community to have a comfortable, secular and, on occasion, even decadent life style. This became a source of concern to those among the friars who took their vows of poverty, chastity, abstinence and obedience seriously. It also aroused the envy of the secular lords who had granted the monks and nuns exclusive brew rights in the first place.

The initial opposition against the secular life style practiced by some of the friars started in the Benedictine abbey of Cluny in Burgundy, founded in 910. It spawned a movement that quickly spread to almost 1,500 affiliated houses all over the realm. The Carthusians at Chartreuse, in the French Alps, started a second monastic revival movement in 1084. The Cistercians at Cîteaux, near Dijon, started a third one in 1098. By the 12th century, a new, purist, anti-secular fervor had taken hold in central Europe and led to a gradual redirection of all facets of monastic life. Once again, piety, poverty and pastoral duties were in, while the secular and profane arts of brewing, commerce and frolicking were out.

In time, the feudal lords, once the benevolent supporters of monastic brewing rights, became increasingly eager to cash in for themselves on the riches that could be gained from the brew industry. They started to create their own court brew houses

(Hofbräuhaus) with exclusive privileges, enforced by the sanctions of the law, over which, of course, they had total control. As a result, many monasteries lost the right to brew commercially, though some retained permission to continue to brew for their own consumption.

One natural, rather than social or political cause, also contributed to the waning of monastic dominance in the brew industry and to the decline of beer consumption in general. This was a climatic accident that occurred in the first few centuries of the second millennium. The earth underwent a warming trend that allowed wine growing to spread rapidly into ever more northern areas. Especially in southern Germany, cheap and plentiful good wine became available and finally rose to become a serious competitor of the once dominant drink from grain. Interestingly, as the monasteries started to lose their beer privileges, they quickly capitalized on the new wave and, once again, became the leaders, both professionally and commercially, in the emerging wine industry and in the production of wine-based distilled spirits and liqueurs.

By the 12th century, feudal aristocrats, especially in southern Germany, began to take over the brew business from the monasteries and convents. A lord would build his own Hofbräuhaus (court brew house) and, if he was charitably inclined, issue a license to a secular private brewery, for a hefty fee, of course, but not always with the desired result. As it turned out, the brewing privileges of the monks and nuns were much more easily transferred than their brewing expertise, and beer quality usually declined. In northern Germany, the story was slightly different. There, forward-looking mercantile entrepreneurs rather than feudal nobles challenged the church for its brew monopoly. The enterprising free burghers usually were fast studies. Eventually they triumphed over the men of the cloth and surpassed them in the quality of the beers they produced.

Emperor Frederick I himself was the author of the first known secular beer regulation in Germany. It dates from 1156 and was part of the first city code of law, the Justitia civitatis Augustensis, which Frederick gave to the city of Augsburg. The emperor decreed that: *"a brewer who makes bad beer or pours an unjust measure shall be punished; his beer shall be destroyed or distributed at no charge among the poor."*

To control the quality (and revenues) of the local suds, the cities started to issue strict and often silly regulations. The tyranny of bureaucracy, in many an instance, replaced the tyranny of aristocracy. In 1293, the city council of Nürnberg tried to improve the beer brewed within its walls by issuing a straightforward ordinance, in which it insisted that only barley be used to brew beer. Other beer ordinances, however, were not so simple or rational. We know of an early, pesky, lengthy and meddlesome ordinance that dates from 1351.

Issued by the magistrate of the city of Erfurt in Thuringia, it states: *"A calibrated tankard must always be filled to the mark. The beer in it shall cost 4½ pfennigs and 8 groschen. No burgher or councilor may brew more than two beers per year, nor may he make half a brew, nor may he mill less or more than three boxes of malt to brew with. Only on Wednesday evening, and not before the beer bell is rung, may he start a fire under the tun and start brewing. But nobody may brew who does not possess containers, tuns, kilns and casks. The beer must be an entire brew. The amount to be brewed must be announced on Walpurgis Day (February 25), and the precise amount announced must then be brewed. Nobody may brew with straw and twigs for fire."*

"Anybody who breaks an innkeeper's beer mug or runs away without paying, will pay a 10-groschen penalty or must leave town. Anybody who buys hops may not touch the measuring jar until the vendor has filled it and has removed his hand from it. (In those days, brewers bought hops by volume, not by weight!) In the countryside, nobody may sell beer from another region nor may he brew without the knowledge of the town. Any burgher caught brewing in the countryside will no longer be considered a burgher of the town."

Here we find an early version of Bierzwang (literally: beer coercion), the parochial practice of the local authorities to permit only those beers to be served within their walls and in the surrounding countryside that were brewed (and taxed) within their own jurisdiction. The Bierzwang remained common in many parts of Germany until 1803, when, under the influence of the Napoleonic conquest of central Europe, Bierfreiheit (beer freedom) was finally established as a matter of law in much of Germany.

In 1250, Regensburg, the town where the Romans had already brewed beer some 1,000 years earlier, received citizen brew privileges from Emperor Frederick II. As business thrived, the brewers found it difficult to resist the temptation to raise their profits by lowering their standards. After a disastrous harvest in 1433 and its resulting grain shortage, the local beer became so scarce that the city fathers permitted the importation of brews from as far away as Hamburg and Dortmund. By 1447, the Regensburgers finally had enough of substandard local brew. They appointed their city doctor, Konrad Megenwart, as the official beer inspector, and, six years later forbade brewers within their city walls to use "seeds, spice, or rushes" as flavorings. (Hellex 1981) To ensure that the citizens would get their money's worth, the city fathers also outlawed the brewing and selling of thin beers made from the final runnings of the mash.

In Munich, too, regulating brewers and their craft was of apparent and perpetual concern to the city fathers of the day, and a clear indication that not all was well with the Bavarians' national beverage. In 1363, to guarantee quality, the 12-member city council itself assumed the duty of overseeing all beer production. By 1372, there were only 21 brewers left in Munich, not even two for every councilor, and the demand of the people for beer kept these brewers so busy that their brew was consumed almost as soon as it was fermented. In 1420, the city fathers tried to decree from above what the market would not do on its own. They insisted that all beers must be aged for at least eight days before they could be sold.

In 1450, the number of brewers had risen to only 30, and the Bavarian ruler, Duke Stephan II, tried to redress the beer shortage by issuing an appeal to his subjects. He implored them to brew more at home so that beer would not be so terribly scarce all the time. It was to take another couple of centuries, before the brewers of southern Germany finally caught up with their northern German brethren. In the 15th century, however, brewing clearly was not an attractive profession in Munich, the city that was destined to become the beer capital of the world.

In areas with an emerging wine industry, the answer to declining beer quality was often sought in outlawing beer making altogether. Such was the case in the Franconian city of Würzburg, where the magistrate, in 1434, after due consultation with the duke and the bishop, forbade brewing "forever." Only three years later, however, the climate of central Europe, which had undergone a warming trend for a few centuries, experienced a sudden reversal. Harsh and long periods of frost decimated almost all the vineyards in southern Germany. Wine had to be imported from south of the Alps, and the price jumped accordingly. Consequently, beer, which had been out of favor with the populace made a quick comeback.

The authorities, however, with the timeless arrogance of the mighty, stubbornly clung to their prohibition ignoring both the popular will and the clandestine brewing that it spawned. But greed, as always, got the better of them and they decided to profit for themselves from what they had so miserably tried to suppress. In 1642, Johann Philipp von Schönborn, the Würzburg duke and bishop himself, started his very own Hofbräuhaus. Thus, in Würzburg, "forever" lasted exactly 208 years. The climatic reversal of 1437 turned out to be long lasting. It brought about a permanent shift in market forces and gave a much-needed boost to the secular brew industry in southern Germany, and, in its wake, spawned even more regulation.

In 1447, the Munich city council issued an ordinance demanding that all brewers use only barley, hops and water for their beers. This was the forerunner of what was to become, half a century later, the famous all-Bavarian beer purity law, the Reinheitsgebot. By 1487, the Bavarian Duke Albrecht IV forced all brewers in the city of Munich to take a public oath of faithful allegiance to the 1447 ordinance. Furthermore, the Duke introduced beer price controls: in winter, a Maß (approximately 1 liter) would cost one silver pfennig, in summer, two. This price difference was to compensate brewers for the extra grain and long storage (lagering) required for stronger summer beers. One of Albrecht's successors, Duke Georg the Rich, in 1493, extended the 1447 ordinance to the duchy of Landshut in central Bavaria. Clearly, a regulatory clean-up was afoot in Bavaria.

The Reinheitsgebot was issued on April 23, 1516. Initially only in feudal Bavaria, but later in all of Germany, it gave government the tools to regulate the ingredients, processes and quality of beer sold to the public. It was drafted by the Bavarian co-rulers Duke Wilhelm IV and Duke Ludwig X and introduced at a meeting of the Assembly of Estates of the Bavarian Realm, at Ingolstadt, some 60 miles north of Munich. The 1516 Reinheitsgebot stipulated that only barley, hops, and water may be used to make the brew. The existence of yeast had not yet been discovered. The Reinheitsgebot is the oldest, still valid food quality law in Germany.

Until the invention of refrigeration in the 1870s, our forebears could not brew what they wanted, but only what nature let them. Only gradually did they gain an empirical, trial-and-error understanding of the factors that influence fermentation. They realized that the ambient temperature in the cellar had something to do with the type of beer they got from the wort. They also noticed that there were two types of fermentation. It would take scientists almost another 300 years to unravel the mystery of these two fermentations. The crafters of the Reinheitsgebot did not know that the key to pure beer was (and still is) the yeast. Yeast are airborne, single-cell fungi that are literally everywhere in the environment. They like to hide out in dank, dark places. The cobwebs in the grain-dust-laden rafters of steamy brew houses made for an ideal yeast habitat. There yeast could idle away its time until luck and a hefty breeze would swish it down into an open fermenter for another sugary meal of sweet wort.

There are two broad families of yeasts that make great beers: ale yeasts and lager yeasts, each with their own very specific thermal comfort zone. Ale yeasts like a cozy, warm environment, somewhere around 59° to 77°F (15° to 25°C), in which they become most active and produce the best-tasting beer, while lager yeasts do their best work, when it is a cool 39° to 48°F (4° to 9°C) or even below. Ale yeasts lose their appetites at lower temperatures and go to sleep, leaving the field for the lager yeasts. Lager yeasts, on the other hand, can still ferment wort at higher temperatures, but then produce off-flavors that tend to be undesirable in beer. Fortunately for the medieval, who had no pure yeast strains to work with, the two yeasts, when present in the same brew, each become dominant in their respective temperature ranges. Both ale and lager yeasts are in suspension in the wort, while they munch their way through the sugars deep inside the fermenter, but only ale yeasts throw up thick, frothy layers of foam at the top of the brew. Ale yeasts, therefore, are also called "top-fermenting". Lager yeasts, by comparison, are much less exuberant surface fermenters and are thus often referred to as "bottom-fermenting." After they have done their job of turning wort into beer, both ale and lager yeasts take a nap (go dormant), and generally sink to the bottom.

Because of the temperature-sensitive nature of yeast, the beer the Reinheitsgebot originally sought to control, was not necessarily a lager. Unbeknown to the medieval brewer, it was probably a lager during the cold Bavarian winters, but it was most certainly an ale in the summer, when demand was greatest.

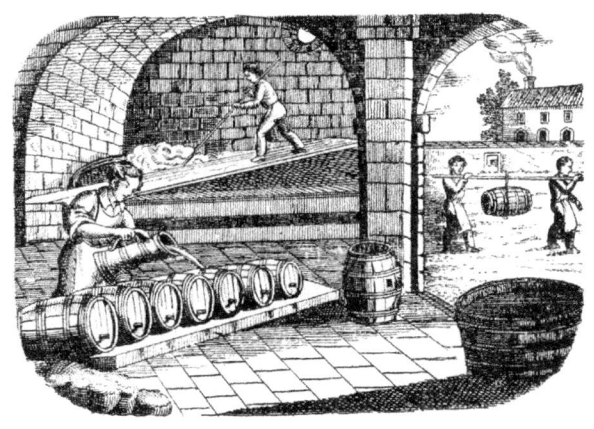

A Munich town council record mentioned cold-fermented beer as early as 1420. Again, in Munich, in 1551, a city ordinance implied that fermentation was not an accidental process but that it could be managed to produce a definite result. It stated that "barley, good hops, water and yeast, if properly mashed and cooled, can also produce a bottom fermenting beer." This is a tantalizing hint at an early awareness of the difference between ales and lagers!

In 1553, summer brewing was outlawed altogether in Bavaria. By then the authorities, always worried about the supply of healthy summer beer, had obviously learned that cold fermentation yielded a purer beer with better keeping qualities than possessed by those unwittingly brewed and probably bacterially infected top-fermented beers of summer. The official brewing season was, therefore, restricted to between St. Michael's Day (September 29) and St. George's Day (April 23). From spring to fall, brewers had to seek alternate employment. It is obvious that this kind of brew schedule, decreed from above, favored the production of lagers. In many breweries, you simply could not make ales in the cold Bavarian winters.

The importance of the two regulations, the Reinheitsgebot and the prohibition against summer brewing, could not be overstated. These laws caused Bavaria to depart from what had been a common German beer culture. They created a north-south schism between a "new" lager culture and the "old" ale culture. Henceforth, Bavarian brewers would chart their own course, moving firmly in the direction of cold-fermented, malted-barley-based lager beers, a style in which, by happenstance and skill, the Bavarians have, some would argue, remained unsurpassed to this day.

By about the 12th century, we observe the birth of a new class of meritorious city burghers linked in trading associations and employing free, wage-earning tradesmen organized in professional guilds. Feudalism, born out of a scarcity of education, money and commerce, in which land and serfs as the only sources of wealth were divided between the learned (the clergy) and the mighty (the lords), soon became an anachronistic shell for a society whose material basis was shifting from land to industry and commerce. Social control over beer making, henceforth, was not so much a struggle between the lord and the monk as one between the lord and the citizen. As the monks and nuns were losing their brew privileges, merchants in the cities, perhaps more faithful to their own fortunes than to God and emperor, knew a good thing when they saw one. They latched on to the brewing trade wherever possible, and soon found themselves in conflict with church and state alike. Especially in northern Germany, where, as a general rule, the hold of church and state over society was less smothering, free merchants, not feudal lords, emerged as the greatest competitors to the cloistered brewers. The worldly merchants opened up new markets by setting up far-flung trading organizations, most famous among them the Hanseatic League, for the exchange of all sorts of goods from spices, to salted fish, to silk, to beer.

The first cracks in the feudal order occurred as early as 924, when King Henry I was forced to build forts and walled towns to protect the eastern flank of his realm against the raids of marauding Magyars. Not getting much help from the noble lords in his fight against the invaders on horseback from the east, the king turned to the ordinary folk and encouraged them to become "burghers" (from the German "Burg" for fort). With this act, Henry had

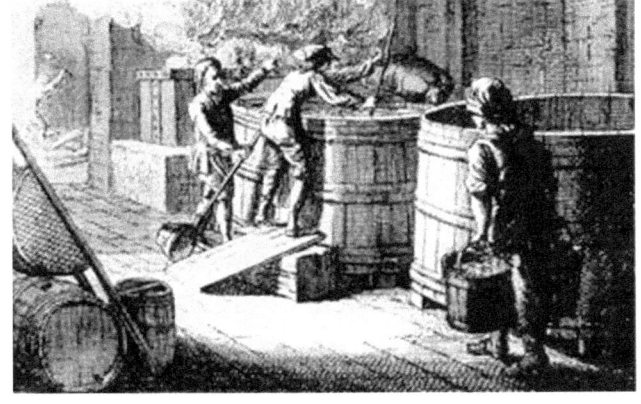

not only created a new word, but an entirely new class. As he built defensive bastions in the frontier regions, he ordered its inhabitants to lay in stores of food for emergencies and to train for combat in marching formations and on horseback. On these burghers, the king also conferred the right to brew beer and to sell it within a mile from the fortifications. These military centers soon became the hubs of judicial, commercial and social activity for the surrounding areas. In these settlements, the new class, the middle class, was, in time, to tear asunder the very foundations of the social order that had evolved in Germany after the collapse of the Roman Empire some five hundred years earlier.

Initially, city brewing, like country brewing, took place only in the home, where it would have stayed had it not been for one problem: In those days, all buildings except for churches, forts and castles were made of wood, and occasionally an entire town would burn down merely because a hausfrau had forgotten to tend the fire under the brew kettle or the bake oven. Many city fathers, therefore, out of concern for public safety, simply forbade home brewing and home baking. They erected communal stone bake-and-brew-houses in which every household had to take turns making its daily bread and beer. Such communal bake and brew facilities created the physical conditions for both the commercialization and the regulation and taxation of city brewing.

As these early city breweries began to hire staff, bakers often doubled as brewers. They already had all the required ingredients on hand. A warm medieval bakehouse was an ideal habitat for airborne yeast cells performing their daily work both as leveners of bread and as fermenters of brew. More often than not, certain yeast strains became dominant in such an environment, as still happens in the rafters and cobwebs of some Belgian lambic houses today, and

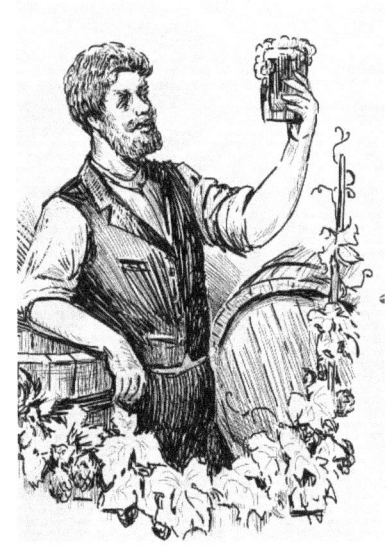 medieval bakers' beers were usually of consistently good quality. Thus, it was only natural that bakers became the local source of both solid and liquid bread and many a city authority gladly granted its bakers the exclusive right to make beer. One fabled such baker-brewer even made it into the Grimm Brothers' early 19th century collection of folk tales (Jacob Grimm 1785-1863; Wilhelm Grimm 1786-1859). Sings Rumpelstiltskin, while he dances around the fire in gleeful anticipation of his blackmail prize, "Today I bake, tomorrow I brew, the day after tomorrow I'll fetch the queen's child."

It was inevitable that, sooner or later, many communal brew houses evolved into real businesses, with inns attached, where artisans and servants could forget the toil of the day over a mug of ale, and where enterprising burghers could congregate to hatch their profitable little deals. Like the monasteries in the countryside, the burgher breweries in the city became thriving businesses, as many a brewpub is today. In time, the interests of the more successful burghers, the patricians of wealth, would collide with those of the feudal holders of power and privilege, including the beer privilege. The feudal lords, whose only claim to fame was that they had been born into the right families, were not part of the cash economy of the entrepreneurs and were eventually reduced to relying on the generosity of the cities for the financing of their wars and their luxurious life style.

One such successful band of medieval burgher entrepreneurs

was the Fugger family of Augsburg. The Fuggers had amassed such wealth through banking and trading in real estate, copper, silver, and mercury that, by the 15th century, they were by far the richest family in Europe. Emperor Maximilian I (1459 - 1519) relied on immense Fugger loans to finance his foreign wars, and in 1519, when it was time to choose Maximilian's successor, the Fuggers secured the election of their man, Charles V, as emperor by bribing the electors. It was Charles V (1500 - 1558), ruler of most of Europe, including Austria and Germany as well as Spain and her colonies around the globe, who could claim, as the first monarch in history, that in his empire "the sun never set," but it was the rising sun of the merchant class that had put him on the throne in the first place. For such support, of course, the titled rulers had to pay a hefty price. They were forced to grant the cities virtual self-government and an ever-increasing share in the government of the realm. In 1521, at the Diet of Worms, Charles conferred upon the city of Augsburg the right to mint its own coins. It is hard to imagine that such favors were not in repayment to the Fugger family of Augsburg to whom he owed so much.

Cities, in effect, became "free". In their charters, they received the right to make laws, mint coins, levy taxes and run their own commercial and political affairs without interference from the nobles. "Stadtluft macht frei" (city air liberates) was the slogan of the burghers, and it enticed many a serf to slip away by night and escape feudal oppression. Where he came from, the serf was owned, literally, by the feudal master, who gave him no other reward for his labors but the rations needed for his family's subsistence. Once in the city, a serf became a free person, who could hire himself out in exchange for wages. He could finally make something of himself.

The burghers made good use of the growing labor pool that was fed from the country side. They organized manufactures, employed the serfs as free craftsmen, established trading networks, and built store houses and retail outlets. Their commercial activities brought ever more wealth and power to the cities, until the might of the cities surpassed that of the official feudal system and its agrarian-based economy. As no-nonsense merchants, the city burghers plied any trade that offered up the promise of profit. And, as the monks and nuns had demonstrated before, one could get rich on beer, especially on top-quality beer. Thus, the most consequential challenge to the brew monopoly of the medieval church came ultimately not from the nobles, but from the rising class of patrician city burghers, especially in northern Germany.

To be sure, there were plenty of arrogant aristocrats and pampered bishops in northern Germany, as there were many enterprising merchant burghers, like the Fugger family, in southern Germany, but, as a general rule, the northerners pursued their aim of civil and economic freedom more aggressively, sometimes even by force of arms, than did their southern counterparts, and, between the 13th and the 16th century, while beer production and beer quality declined in the south, beer became mostly a northern German affair.

The city burghers and their councils had gained virtual control over the brewing industry within their walls by the end of the 12th century. Like the nobles before them, city governments often declared that they alone owned the exclusive right to brew. The nobles, harkening back to a world order that was no more, were powerless to stop them.

By the 13th century, many merchants had fully understood that the feudal state could no longer adequately protect their interests at home or abroad. Especially in the towns involved in trade with the Baltic lands, civic associations and merchant guilds joined forces to form trading leagues. The merchants of Bremen and Hamburg, for instance, set up a joint representation in Novgorod, Russia, to deal with the Czar.

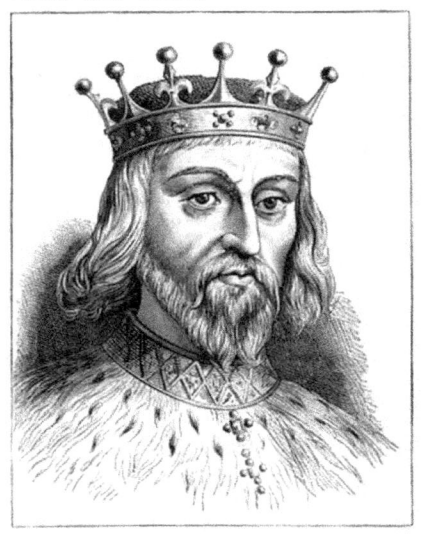

In London, King Henry II granted German city merchants special licenses and privileges as early as 1157. He even gave them a special residence, a guild hall, later to be called the Steelyard House on the Thames. In 1194, King Richard I granted the Steelyard merchants from Cologne freedom from all tolls and customs in London and the right to trade at fairs throughout England. These rights were later extended to the other members of the Steelyard. Soon, the Steelyard became a whole, walled-in community, with its own warehouses, weigh house, church, offices and residential quarters. It spawned affiliated houses in many other English ports.

Political impotence within the Holy Roman Empire of the German Nation as well as difficulties experienced by its seafaring merchants from pirates, feudal regulations against foreign trade, and excessive customs, fostered an ever-closer union among the leading German trading cities. In 1241, Lübeck and Hamburg, on either side of the Danish Peninsula, concluded a treaty of mutual protection, a patrician alliance. In 1266, King Henry III of England gave the Steelyard merchants of Hamburg and Lübeck their own, separate charter, making them the most powerful merchant colony in London.

Other German cities soon joined the protective association of Hamburg and Lübeck, and a strong formal alliance, the Hanseatic League, grew up among them, with Lübeck, the center of the Baltic trade, as its hub. The League eventually included some 200 cities. It fought and won its own wars, as, for instance, in 1368 - 1369, against the Danish King Waldemar IV, whose countrymen, reminiscent of Viking times, had taken to piracy and helped themselves regularly to "free" beer from the League's freighters. The League signed its own peace treaties with foreign governments. One such was the Treaty of Stralsund (1370), which gave it a virtual trade monopoly in all of Scandinavia. Henceforth, no Danish king could be crowned without the League's formal approval.

The League traded in almost any type of commodity, including wine, oil, grain, leather, cloth, copper, iron, salt and beer. Thanks to the League, a consumer could buy Polish mustard in England, Turkish raisins in Flanders, Italian figs in Norway, and German beer in Russia. By cutting out the feudals, the League had created, in effect, the first European common market, free of tariffs and artificial trade restrictions.

Not just port cities like Bremen, Hamburg and Lübeck were part of the Hanseatic League. Cities further inland, such as Einbeck, Brunswick, Breslau, Magdeburg, Dortmund, and Cologne, too, were eager to join the new network and supply the growing trading empire with goods, of which beer became one of the more important export commodities.

Soon wagon loads of export brews would rumble down the dusty northern highways on their way to the harbor storehouses of the Hanseatic merchants. Bremen took the early lead in beer exports sending casks of German ale as far as Flanders, England and Scandinavia. The Brunswick Mumme, a brown, very hoppy barley ale was so strong that it remained palatable almost forever and made its way on sailing ships around to globe, even to the hot East Indies. The golden age of the beer trade was made possible not only by the ever increasing keeping qualities of the northern beers, but also by momentous advances in animal traction and harness. Improvements in these fields were first reported in the ninth century, but came into wider use only around the 13th century.

Before that time, a horse was hitched to its dray by traces fastened to a yoke on its withers and anchored by a strap around the breast. The harder the horse pulled, the more the strap choked it. The rigid collar changed all that. It put the strain on the horse's shoulders instead on its windpipe, thus increasing the animal's "horsepower" almost fivefold. Only then began the transport of heavy casks of beer over rutty roads, as it was now possible. Horses employed in freight hauling were also susceptible to slipping, hoof breakage and foot injuries. Because of frequent breakdowns of the hey burners, delivery schedules for trading goods were notoriously unreliable. It was not until the arrival of the nailed-on, iron horseshoe, which kept the animals sound and sure-footed, that trade, especially in semi-perishable goods, could be conducted on anything resembling a time table.

Another Hanseatic city that had been thriving on beer since the middle of the 13th century was Einbeck. Early users of hops instead of gruit, Einbecker brewers made a strong, cold-conditioned brown ale from barley and wheat, not unlike today's Alt, with excellent keeping properties. Eventually, there would be several hundred breweries in Einbeck, all strictly regulated, and taxed, by the city fathers. Einbeckers shipped their brew by wagon trains to Hamburg,

Bremen and Lübeck, from where it sailed in the holds of Hanseatic ketches to places like Amsterdam to the west and Reval to the east, and even to Jerusalem, where it may have quenched the thirst of a crusading knight.

Perhaps the most important destination of Einbecker beer, at least from hindsight, was Munich. Bavarians who could afford it, especially the nobles, would drink the ale from Einbeck before they would swig the lower-quality local brew. The Bavarian answer to the competition was twofold. They issued the Reinheitsgebot and started to imitate the northern brews locally, but, at first, to no avail. The imports from the north kept on coming. They remained the most popular drink in Munich, and, by 1569, there were still only 53 small breweries in the entire city.

The beers from the north were good, but expensive and a constant drain on Bavaria's money supply, much to the chagrin of Duke Wilhelm V. He ran his own brew house in Landshut, where, in 1590, he had a new beer brewed, a strong brown to red lager, which he hoped would finally recapture the market lost to the northern brewers. A year later, he completed a new brew house in Munich, on the site of the now famous Hofbräuhaus. By 1610, that Munich court brew house made its first deliveries to local innkeepers and private households.

But it was Wilhelm V's successor, Maximilian I, who landed a grand coup that finally spelled an end to the dominance of northern beers in Munich. In 1612, he enticed one Einbecker brew master, Elias Pichler, to come to Munich and create an authentic copy of the famous original Einbecker beer. Once there, poor Elias was not allowed to leave town for purpose or pleasure. He had become too valuable a state asset to be allowed to run free. The Bavarian dialect soon mangled the name Einbeck to ayn pock and, eventually, to ein Bock. The beer itself metamorphosed, under Bavarian influence, from a strong ale into a strong lager, which is what we know as Bock beer today.

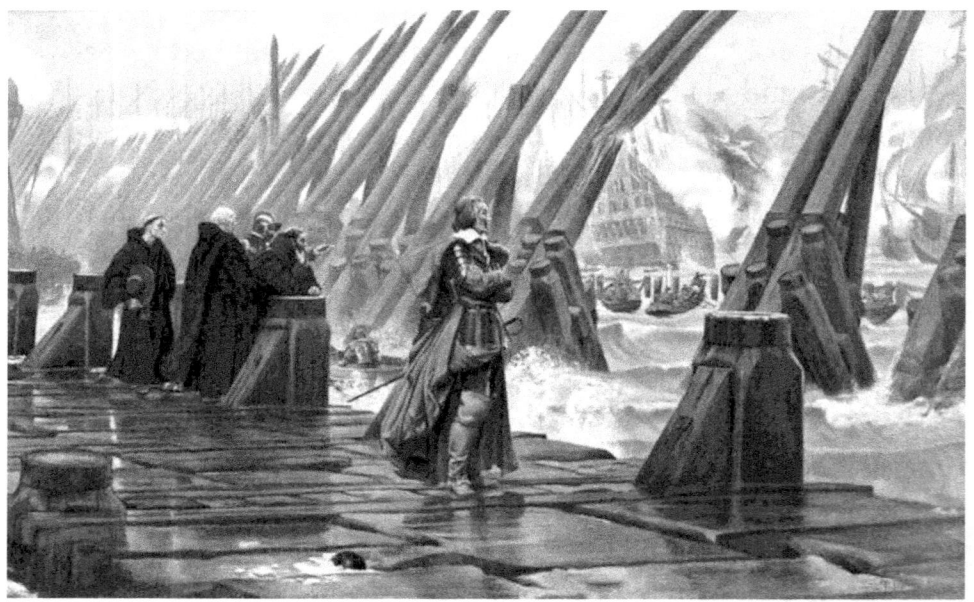

The popularity of Elias' beer became so great that Maximilian was able to finance most of his military expenditures during the Thirty Year's War out of the revenues from the brown lager made by this transplanted brew master. Bavaria was finally on its way to becoming the beer stronghold it is today.

As more and more beer passed through the Hanseatic port city of Bremen, its merchant burghers soon figured that they could make more money by making the beer themselves instead of just buying it from others and trading in it. By the end of the 13th century, thanks to the skills of Bremer brewers and to the sheer size of the markets of the Hanseatic League, no beer was more popular and plentiful in

Europe than that brewed in Bremen.

The Hamburgers, too, soon entered the international beer business and, during the 14th century, started to eclipse their rivals from Bremen. Hamburg emerged as the brewing city of the League, though Bremen continued to be the premier export harbor for beers from Einbeck, Göttingen and Brunswick. By 1376, Hamburg recorded 457 burgher-owned breweries, by 1526 there were 531. Together, they brewed almost 25 million liters per year (more than 200,000 barrels) and employed almost half the city's wage earning population. Their most famous brew was Keutebier, a hopped, reddish to dark-brown wheat beer with an up-front sweetness and a viniferous aftertaste.

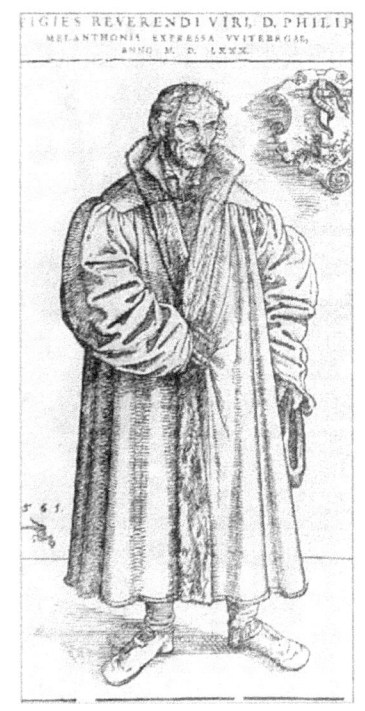

One of the more ardent lovers of Hamburg beer was Luther's reformer cohort and confidant, Philipp Melanchton. Even on his death bed, in Wittenberg, in 1560, Philipp asked for a bowl of beer soup. Knowing that it would be his last meal, he specified that it be made with Hamburg suds. How is that for brand loyalty?

The Hannoverians developed their own version of a wheat ale, the Broyhan beer, so-named after Cord Broyhan, a Hannoverian native who had left his home town to apprentice with a Hamburg brewer. There he learned the secrets of Hamburger beer. When he returned home, in 1526, he started his own brewery and made his variation on the Hamburg theme, a well-hopped, light brown ale, mashed from one third wheat and two thirds barley.

Soon other entrepreneurs jumped on the Broyhan bandwagon. In 1609, the city council of Hannover regulated the quality and brew techniques of the local Broyhan beer, limited the number of brewer burghers to 317, combined all of them into one guild, and incorporated the guild as a company. The guild brewery still exists today as a stock holders' company and is the oldest enterprise in Hannover.

It was the Thirty Year's War that was the death knell of the Hanseatic League and, with it, the glory of northern brewing. After the war's disruptive turmoil, which pitted the Protestant against the Catholic countries of Europe, Germany was devastated. Its cities were plundered, its fields lay fallow, its soil was blood-soaked, its commerce was at a standstill, and the Holy Roman Empire was reduced to a mere shell of its former greatness. Many monasteries and feudal castles lay in ruin as did their breweries, never to be rebuilt. Germany was split into 370 semi-autonomous states and statelettes, all with their own trade restrictions and with borders and customs duties that made trade all but impossible.

The Hanseatic League formally dissolved in 1669, but its lasting legacy was a change in the economic balance of power in Europe away from the landed feudals to the city-dwelling bourgeoisie. In its wake, the war left behind a vacuum waiting to be filled by new social organizations and a new, more liberated mindset with an openness to new ideas that would bring progress in all facets of life.

The old feudal rulers of the Dutchy of Bavaria, the House of Wittelsbach, came to power in 1180. Whatever their political fortunes, as guardians of their subjects' beer, they have a lot to answer for. For the first 300 years of their reign, they tried to keep the brewing of ales and lagers, and the profits that came with it, out of the hands of the monks and the burghers and reserved it for themselves and their cronies. Then, for the next 100 years or so, they almost wiped out ale brewing by passing regulations that favored lager making in general and strengthened the market position of their own court breweries in particular. In the end, though, they reinstated ale making, but only as wheat beer, and monopolized it completely, after it became clear how much money they could make from it.

Today, when we think of ales, we picture in our mind a beer that is hearty, full bodied, satisfying, nourishing and substantial. When we think of lagers, by comparison, we picture a beer that is delicate, subtle, dainty and gentile. Not so in the Bavaria of the 16th century. After the beer purity law of 1516 (the Reinheitsgebot) and the summer brew prohibition of 1553, barley-based lagers were brown and smoky, while wheat-based ales were "white beers" (Weissbier) that were crisp and delicious.

In Bavaria, as in the rest of Germany, any grain was acceptable for beer brewing, the Wittelsbacher co-dukes Wilhelm IV and Ludwig X, proclaimed that wheat would not make "pure" beer. That assertion must have been a kick in the teeth for the Degenberg clan, a noble family from the village of Schwarzach, near Munich, which had been brewing wheat ales for decades. The Degenbergers considered themselves the sole owners of the privilege to make and sell the brew in Bavaria.

The notable omission by the dukes of wheat as a legitimate raw material for beer in the original Reinheitsgebot is probably no accident, but a combination of vanity, paternalism, politics and fiscal avarice. The dukes considered Weissbier too gentile a beverage for the vulgar masses, for whom the brown lagers of the time were deemed good enough, especially, after the dukes had decreed that they be pure.

Also, there were frequent wheat shortages in medieval Bavaria, and the dukes, well-acquainted with their subjects' nefarious habits, feared that the good Bavarians would rather forego their daily bread than not have their daily brew. Since it was the God-given duty of the feudal lords to look after the welfare of their subjects, they held, in their paternal wisdom, that wheat would best serve the common good if it were consumed in solid rather than liquid form. The dukes considered wheat beer "a useless drink that neither nourishes nor provides strength and power, but only encourages drunkenness" unless, of course, it was destined to slacken a noble thirst! By 1566, fifty years after the Reinheitsgebot, wheat beer making by the ordinary brewer was outlawed altogether.

On the political side, the dukes had to respect the inherited monopoly of wheat beer brewing enjoyed by the House of Degenberg. Blatant revocation of a feudal privilege was unthinkable in an era when the power of the state to make war depended on the willingness of the landed gentry to supply the infantry with serfs. The local lords, who owned the serfs, traded the military services of their subjects for rights and privileges. They usually drove a hard bargain, exacting advantages for themselves in perpetuity.

While Wilhelm IV confirmed and even extended the Degenbergers' right to brew and sell Weissbier, his successor, Duke Abrecht V, however, was not so generous. He tried to make life and business as difficult as possible for the Degenbergers by putting a sales tax on their suds, thus provoking a feud between the two houses, the Wittelsbachers and the Degenbergers, that lasted until 1602. In that auspicious year, happily for the dukes, the line of Degenbergers became extinct, when its last progeny, Baron Hans Sigmund of Degenberg, died without leaving an heir. By the rules of the day, the wheat beer privilege automatically reverted to the house of the Bavarian dukes.

Now that the dukes, instead of the Degenbergers, could make money from wheat beer, there was a sudden reversal of official Bavarian policy. Duke Maximilian I, great-grandson of Wilhelm IV, of Reinheitsgebot fame, built a new court brew house in Munich, right next to the brown lager brewery built by his father Wilhelm V. Both breweries were, incidentally, on the site of the now-famous Munich Hofbräuhaus at Am Platzl Square.

Maximilian I brought the Schwarzach brew master to Munich and dedicated the new brewery exclusively to Weissbier making. Over the years, he added more and more wheat beer breweries to his brew conglomerate. He also continued to prevent anybody else from brewing wheat beers and, thus, granted to the line of Wittelsbachers the only exception from the barley-only provisions of the Reinheitsgebot.

Not only was wheat beer now permitted to be dispensed to the masses, in fact, every innkeeper had to pour it, next to the standard brown lager, and purchase it directly from the crown! If he refused, he lost his license. This new twist in Bavarian beer policy not only kept the wheat beer flowing in the land but also the coffers swelling in the ducal treasury.

The Weissbier monopoly remained with the Wittelsbachers until well into the 19th century, by which time the Bavarian rulers had earned sheer astronomical sums from the sale to the humble masses of the erstwhile upper crust quaff. They even issued a wheat beer quality ordinance, in 1803, in which they specified that the brew should:

"be bubbly and foamy, contain the bitterness of the hops, leave a cooling and refreshing sensation on the palate, and impart its prickly flavor to its bouquet as well."

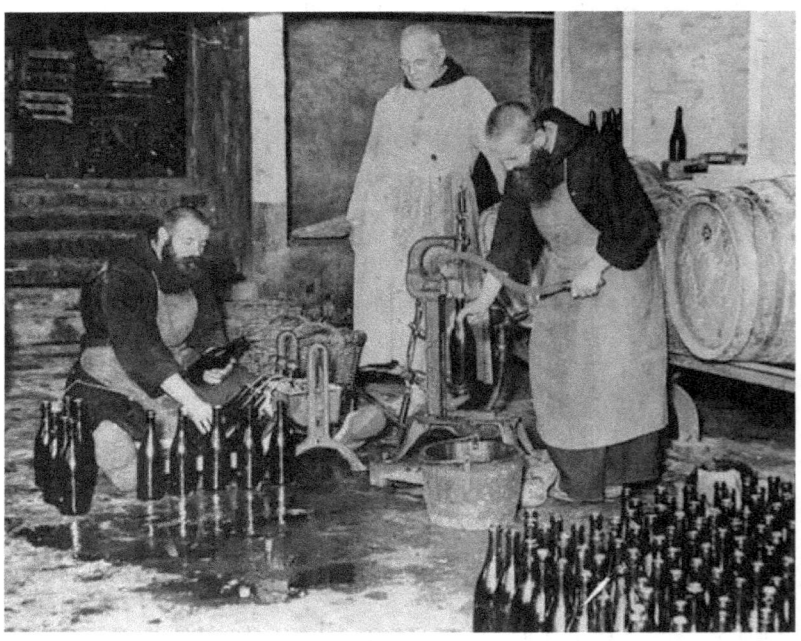

Thus, in spite of the Reinheitsgebot, which put lagers on the map, Bavaria became the cradle of German wheat ale, by decree from above, not by democratic market forces from below... simply because there was money in it for the nobles.

Eventually, though, the brown lager of Bavaria improved and made a comeback. By 1808, the ducal brown beer brewery incorporated the adjacent wheat beer brewery into its operations. By the mid-1800s, wheat beers had become just a curiosity from the past. In 1872, the Wittelsbachers sold the Weissbier privilege to a private brewing company and thus ended two-and-a-half centuries of the ducal wheat beer monopoly. In the decades that followed, wheat beer sales stabilized.

Though the Reinheitsgebot has changed in modern times and now allows for malted wheat in certain beers, the Weissbier has not. It's still an ale. There is no lager wheat beer in Germany. It would be against the law! All beers called Weizen or Weissbier must be made with top-fermenting yeast and at least 50 percent malted wheat. Furthermore, the addition of unmalted wheat--or unmalted anything, for that matter--is verboten.

Today, dozens of private breweries turn out wheat ale in all shades of color and alcoholic strength--from clear, blond, filtered Kristallweizen, to pale, unfiltered Hefeweizen, to dark Dunkelweizen, to strong Weizenbock and even Weizendoppelbock. Ale made from wheat now comprise a some 10 percent of German beer consumption and is available in stores and pubs across the country from Hamburg to Munich, from Düsseldorf to Dresden.

Even after the demise of the Hanseatic League and the stagnation of the brew industry in the north, free brewing continued in Germany. In Bavaria, monastery and court breweries were being replaced by commercial ones. While between the 12th and 16th century, much of the top-quality brew consumed in Bavaria had to be imported from northern Germany, by 1750, some 4,000, mostly very small, commercial breweries had sprung up in Bavaria, all making excellent, mostly lager, beer. Every little village and hamlet had its own brewery, usually protected by local monopoly ordinances and supplying its tiny patch of the universe with brew.

In some areas in Bavaria, the prohibition against drinking beer from another town remained in force until about 200 years ago.

The political and economic victory of the bourgeoisie ultimately proved lasting, even in Bavaria. After the French Revolution (1789), rumblings of freedom were heard even in the most staunchly conservative and reactionary regions of Europe. In 1797, the French, imbued with democratic fervor, occupied the Rhineland, including Düsseldorf and Cologne. By 1806, Napoleon Bonaparte ruled most of Europe. In that year, the German Emperor, Francis II, who was also the king of Austria, resigned, and the Holy Roman Empire of the German Nation, which Otto I had founded in 962, was formally dissolved. According to Francis II, it was no longer worth governing.

In an effort to maintain social control of the conquered Rhineland, the newly-instated governor and brother-in-law to Napoleon, Joaquim Murat, forbade all trade and professional associations. This was the end of the brewer's guilds in Düsseldorf, Cologne and most anywhere else in Germany.

Even in Bavaria, in the year 1800, local beer sale monopolies were abolished and every subject was allowed to drink whichever beer he wanted, even if it was from the next town instead of the local brewery. After 1805, country breweries were allowed to brew as much beer as their city competitors, and all breweries could own and operate brewpubs.

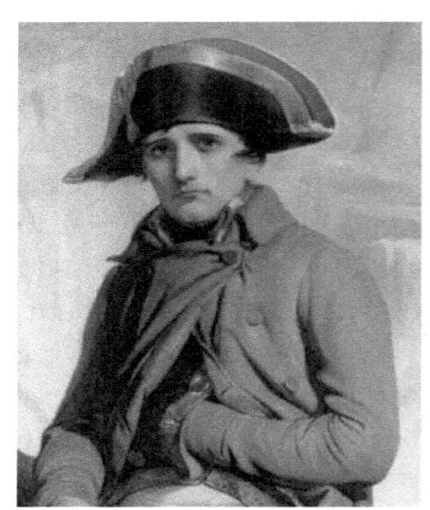

After the defeat of Napoleon at

Waterloo (1815) and the peace treaty hammered out during the Vienna Congress that same year, the Rhineland became a province of Prussia. The Prussian rulers confirmed the abolition of the guilds, arguing that their rules of admission had been too restrictive. Henceforth, there was to be Gewerbefreiheit, the freedom of every Prussian subject to choose his own profession or trade, unhampered by the closed-shop restrictions of the guilds. In the early 19th century, protectionism in the beer business slowly fell by the wayside and competition became the rule. Brewing in most parts of Germany had become unshackled from its traditional limitations, except taxes, of course, and had been tossed into the treacherous waters of the open market. In Munich, for instance, in 1790, there were 60 breweries supplying the city's 40,000 inhabitants. By 1819, there were only 35 left, and by 1865, no more than 15. The market place eliminated inefficient enterprises, but those that survived the shake-out became bigger. Freed from the constraints of religious dogma and feudal backwardness, critical free thought and scientific inquiry also took off. The changes in the intellectual world had started in the 17th century, after the Thirty Years' War, and had a profound impact on beer and brewing.

Since Sumerian and Egyptian times, beer had been made by spontaneous, uncontrolled fermentation. The ancients dropped a loaf of half-baked bread into a jar filled with water. They waited a few days, then took a straw and imbibed.

The monks, nuns, vassals, housewives and craftsmen of the Middle Ages refined the techniques, but still had no clue which processes they actually set in motion. The result of their efforts was, more often than not, an ale, rarely a lager, but always chancy. Only with the rise of commercial freedom, intellectual enlightenment, and science and technology could beer making reach new heights. It was not until the 19th century that beer began to taste reliably and ubiquitously good. To reach the level of proficiency of a modern brewer, man had to figure out what actually happened in the fermenter. Man, needed to see, to understand and to control. That development took roughly from the start of the 17th to the end of the 19th century. It was driven by discovery and innovation, and, within the span of a scant 250 years, man moved from brewing by the seats of his pants to a scientific understanding and to technological control of the processes required for beer quality and consistency.

Until the 16th century, government regulations like the Reinheitsgebot and the summer brewing prohibition were the driving forces behind the changes in brewing practices, particularly in Bavaria. But even after 1516, when only barley, hops and water were used, the result of the brewing process was still a matter of luck. Fermentation was commonly regarded as a mystical and spontaneous process, a form of putrefaction. The milky substance that settled out at the bottom of the fermenter or formed a flocculent layer at the top of the brew was not recognized for what it was (yeast). Instead, it was considered an impurity, a by-product of putrefaction that better be discarded. It was not known that this very "by-product" made alcoholic fermentation happen.

In practice, any number of airborne yeast strains, from lager yeasts (saccharomyces uvarum) to ale yeasts (saccharomyces cerevisiae) to wild yeasts, could be, and probably were present in any given brew and, most likely, all were infected with bacteria. Which yeast became dominant and defined the character of the beer depended largely on the ambient temperature. The warmer the cellar, the more likely the beer would be an ale. Off-flavors in beer and a short shelf life were probably the rule rather than the exception, especially for beers brewed during hot summer months.

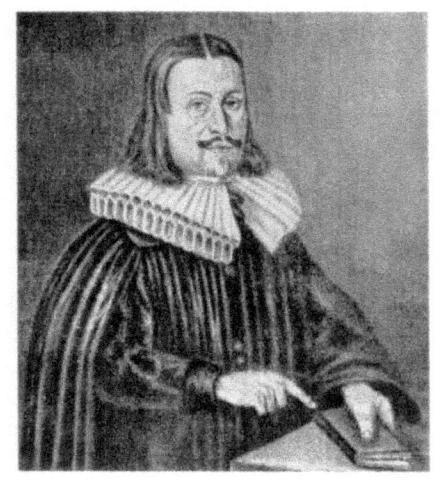

A theoretical understanding of the metabolism of yeast, of the differences between warm and cold fermenting yeasts, and of the differences between the beers they produce, had to wait until the late 19th century.

It was the German physician and chemist Andreas Libau, a.k.a. Libavius (sometime around 1590), who was the first to point out that fermentation and putrefaction were different processes. He knew about carbon dioxide (CO_2) and was the first to describe a method of distilling alcohol. It is doubtful that any brewer of Libavius' time read his heavy tome, *Alchymia* (published in Latin, in 1606), which was the first systematic text book of chemistry, but later scientists did. Libavius laid the conceptual foundation for all subsequent discoveries about the true nature of fermentation.

The Thirty Years' War had not only devastated central Europe physically, it also had brought most scientific work to a halt. Progress started to pick up only towards the 18th century, when the Age of Reason ushered in a new wave of intellectual, political, social and economic change and propelled the Western world towards democracy, industrialization and a much more secular lifestyle.

Although Antony van Leeuwenhoek (1632-1723) appears to have had no interest in brewing, he was, without realizing it, the instrument for the research that would ultimately solve the mystery of fermentation. Van Leeuwenhoek was a draper-turned-natural-scientist-and-microscope-maker. As a draper apprentice in

Amsterdam, in 1648, young Antony often had to check the quality of cloth under a lens. This helped spark his interest in optics. By 1871, he had constructed his first microscope. He assembled at least 242 of them in his lifetime, some with a magnification of as great as 270 times.

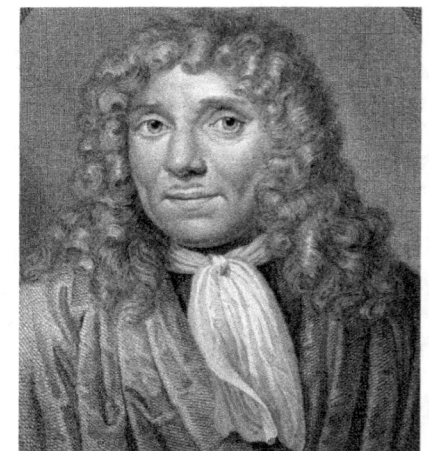

We know that Zacharias Janssen, a Dutch spectacle maker, had theorized about magnification before van Leeuwenhoek and had made a primitive model of the microscope around 1590 (as had Galileo in 1610), but van Leeuwenhoek's was the first truly usable device. In 1674, it helped him to see yeast cells, bacteria, and other protozoa (single-cell animals) as well as red blood cells for the very first time. He also described the reproduction of microorganisms and thus refuted the theory of spontaneous generation, which, thus far, had furnished the accepted explanation for the cause of fermentation and putrefaction.

Finally, there was the yeast! Have you ever thought what brewing would be like without a thermometer or even a clock? The invention of the first mechanical clock is credited to a learned monk, Gerbert, who later became Pope Sylvester II. His contraption dates from around 996 AD, but mechanical clocks did not come into wider use until the late Middle Ages. Imagine controlling the mashing time or the boil in the brew kettle by keeping a watchful eye on an hourglass or maybe a sundial. Great variation in extract efficiency and beer quality must have been the order of the day, when time was more a matter of guesswork than measurement.

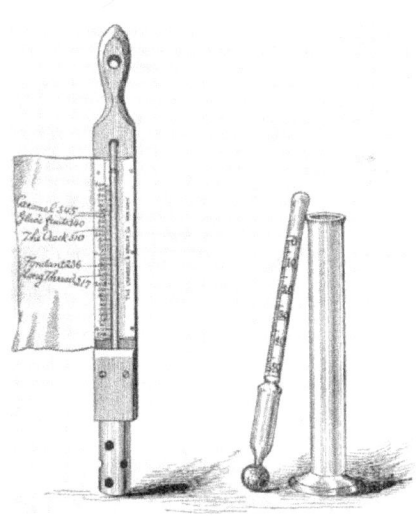

The thermometer was not invented until a mere 250 years ago, the first usable thermometers were developed by a German named Gabriel Daniel Fahrenheit, in 1714, by a Frenchman named René Antoine Ferchault de Réaumur, in 1731, and by a Swede named Anders Celsius, in 1742. This new little gadget finally allowed brewers to control mash temperatures without having to mix fixed volumes of grain and water at either well water temperature or at a boil.

The French chemist Antoine Laurent Lavoisier (1743 - 1794) made the next giant leap forward in fermentation knowledge. In 1789, he discovered that CO_2 and ethanol are the products of alcoholic fermentation. He also explained the role of oxygen in the respiration of both plants and animals and thus contributed to our understanding of the carbon cycle that turns the barley on the stalk into the brew in our glass. After 1818, the taste of beer improved greatly as indirect hot-air kilning of malted grain gradually replaced the traditional direct-smoke kilning. Instead of sending hot, dirty smoke over the moist bed of malted grain, in an indirect system, the fuel heated a stream of clean air that was blown through the grain. Thus, the grain no longer picked up smoky residues from coal or wood, flavors that used to be passed on to the beer. The new kilns also allowed for more precise temperature control of the drying grain and thus gave the brewer, for the first time, dependable pale malt as well as malt with predictable mashing qualities.

By the beginning of the 19th century brewers knew that fermentation had nothing to do with rot, that yeast played an important role, and, thanks to Lavoisier, that fermentation produced alcohol and CO_2. Now it was time for someone to put it all together and to explain the mechanisms at work in detail. Along came the German physiologist and histologist Theodor Schwann (1810 - 1882). Schwann discovered that the cell is the building block of all plant and animal tissue. He was also the first to recognize, in 1837, that the yeast cell, which was first seen by van Leeuwenhoek under his microscope, is a living organism. Noting that the little critter had a sweet tooth, he called it "sugar fungus," hence the Latin name *saccharomyces*. Schwann also discovered that the munching of sugars by *saccharomyces*, which we call fermentation, occurs only when there is no air, i.e. that fermentation is an anaerobic process.

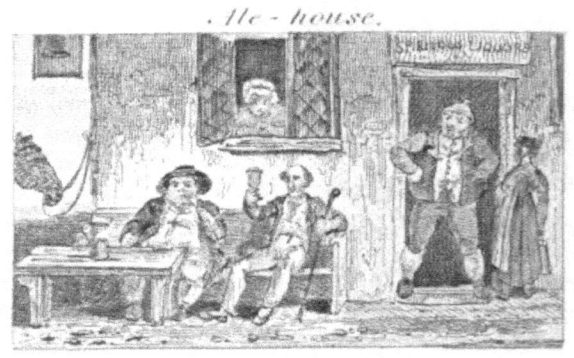

In 1843, only one year after the first Pilsner Urquell was brewed, the Bohemian chemist Carl Joseph Napoleon Balling invented the hydrometer. His gravity spindle measured the amount of dissolved substances in the wort, mostly sugars, but also proteins, minerals, vitamins and aromatics, and thus allowed for the quantitative determination of extract strength and of the progress of fermentation (which brewers call attenuation). Brewing science was finally getting somewhere! The milky by-product of medieval putrefaction had by now become firmly established as a living, single-cell creature that converted sugars into alcohol and carbon dioxide and thus turns the brewer's wort into beer. Brewers could control the color of the grain that they fed the yeast, they could measure the yeast's temperature while it was at work in order to predict if they were producing a lager or an ale, and they could check the progress of the yeast's labors with a hydrometer. But if they wanted to tame the yeast, they had to find out what made it tick. The French chemist Louis Pasteur was the one to furnish that answer.

Louis Pasteur (1822 - 1895) became interested in the fermentation of wine, vinegar and beer while he was a professor at universities in Dijon, Strasbourg and Lille. By 1862, we find him at the École normale in Paris, where he was poised to finished off the myth of spontaneous fermentation for good. He discovered that heating liquids to about 145°F for 30 minutes kills any bacteria or other organisms that it may contain (today we call this pasteurization), and that, if the liquid is left hermetically sealed, no microbial activity, spontaneous or otherwise, recurs. Always eager to increase the shelf life of their beers, breweries were among the first industries to pasteurize their products.

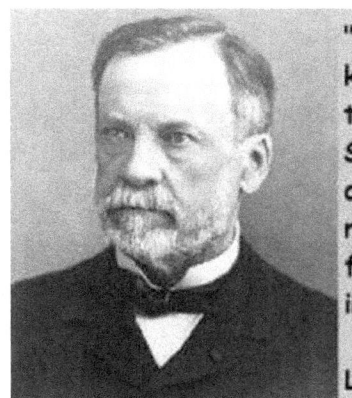

"Science knows no country, because knowledge belongs to humanity, and is the torch which illuminates the world. Science is the highest personification of the nation because that nation will remain the first which carries the furthest the works of thought and intelligence."

Louis Pasteur

Since infectants cannot suddenly appear in a sterile environment, but must be introduced from the outside, Pasteur also admonished brewers to examine yeast cells under the microscope before adding them to the beer (pitching) in order to determine whether the yeast was infected or healthy.

In 1868, Pasteur moved to the Sorbonne. Two years later, he was commissioned by the French government to investigate how French brewers could make a beer that could compete effectively against the rising flood of imports from Germany. Eight years later, he spelled out his findings in his study *Études sur la bière*, which did not rescue the French beer market from domination by the neighboring Teutonic brew, but did provide the most comprehensive explanation yet of the fermentation processes and the products that result from the yeast's metabolism.

He discovered that yeast metabolizes glucose (a type of sugar) under the presence of oxygen and that it uses energy gained from the sugar to grow and reproduce furiously. Under anaerobic conditions, yeast does not grow much, but, as Schwann had already observed, commences vigorous fermentation. This rule is now known as the Pasteur effect: Oxygen suppresses fermentation, its absence stimulates it.

Since Pasteur, we can manage the metabolic life of yeast through wort aeration after pitching and through subsequent oxygen starvation. We also know that, if we start out with sterile wort and control the microbes we pitch into the brew, we can control the result and make good beer. Thanks to Pasteur, hygiene has become one of the most important tools in the brewer's repertoire.

What was still needed was a practical way to segregate the different yeast strains and breed them pure. This problem was solved by the Danish botanist Emil Christian Hansen (1842 - 1909), a recognized authority on fungi (myces). From 1879, Hansen worked as head of the laboratory of the Carlsberg Brewing Company in Copenhagen.

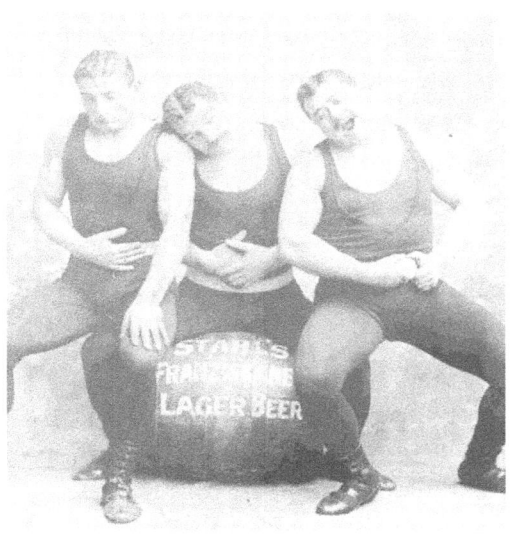

He was the first, in 1881, to classify brewer's yeast into cold, bottom-fermenting lager strains (*saccharomyces uvarum*) and warm, top fermenting ale strains (*saccharomyces cerevisiae*). All other yeasts are called "wild" in beer making and produce nasty off-flavors. *Saccharomyces uvarum*, incidentally, is also known as *saccharomyces Carlsbergensis*. It is not difficult to figure out where that name comes from. Hansen also noted that, within the two broad classes of beer-friendly top and bottom fermenting yeasts, there are many variations, each with their own properties that affect the ultimate taste of the beer they ferment. Already in 1882, he demanded that yeast not only be free from bacteria, as Pasteur had insisted, but also free from "wild" yeast, if we want to make good beer. By 1890, he had developed a practical technique for the cultivation of pure yeast strains from a single cell. Pitching was never to be the same again.

The British chemist Cornelius O'Sullivan was the first to figure out how enzymes work. As biochemical catalysts, enzymes convert, under the influence of moisture and warmth, unfermentable starches into fermentable sugars. O'Sullivan published his findings in 1890 and, thus, demystified the riddle of the mash. He supplied us with the last missing link in our understanding of the carbon chain from the carbon dioxide in the air, to the starch in the grain, to the sugar in the wort, to the alcohol in the fermented beer. We now had the biochemistry of both lager and ale fermentation under control. But its practical application year-round still required a better way of controlling fermentation temperatures. By the middle of the 19th century, it was clearly understood that yeast works best only in a very narrow temperature range. Only then does it make beer with a good flavor. It was the invention of a German engineer, Carl von Linde, that finally allowed brewers to replace the traditional ice houses with mechanical refrigeration. The breakthrough came in 1873, when Linde, with the financial backing of Gabriel Sedlmayr, brew master at the Munich Spaten Brewery, completed his first working model of what was then called an ammonia cold machine.

Linde recognized that a compressed gas when it is permitted to expand, or a solid when it is liquefied, absorbs heat from its surroundings. Ammonia, CO2, freon, or several other volatile chemicals can be used as refrigerants, as long as they lend themselves to alternating condensation and evaporation in a closed system. Linde used an electromotor to compress gaseous ammonia into a liquid. He then released it into the coils of a refrigeration compartment. There the ammonia reverted to its gaseous form and, in the process, drew heat from its environment. The motor then repeated the cycle by converting the ammonia gas back into a liquid, and so on and so on. Compression is best done away from the refrigerated area, because compression gives off heat.

Depending on the sources, different people, including Linde, have been credited with the invention of refrigeration, but it was Linde's work with the new technology and the enthusiastic support of brew master Sedlmayr that led to the universal embrace of refrigeration by the brewing industry. To this day, the compressors and evaporators in a modern brewery still work according to the same principles that Linde used in his first cold machine. In 1878,

Lorenz Enzinger, a Bavarian living in Worms, on the banks of the Rhine river, brought a filtration device on the market that took yeast and other suspended solids out of the beer before it was packaged. This gave beer clarity and a longer shelf life. Two years later, the first patented machine for dispensing beer with CO_2 instead of air appeared. Now even draft beer stayed fresh to the last drop.

Advances in such areas as water chemistry, grain and hops botany, metallurgy, thermodynamics and packaging technology all contributed to enhancements in the quality of beer. Grain botany gave us laboratory-bred barley of high enzymatic power, low levels of protein, and a minimum of resinous and phenolic off-flavors. Hop breeders developed varieties with specific bittering (alpha-acid) ranges and aroma oils. Improved malting techniques gave us better control over beer color and flavor, and the enzymatic properties of brewing grains. New mash tun, brew kettle and fermenter designs allowed for perfect temperature control, high extract efficiency, and wort sterility.

While most of the developments described above benefited the quality of both ales and lagers, it was Hansen's and Linde's pioneering work, which occurred only a little more than a hundred years ago, that made the modern lager revolution possible. As we have seen, brewers certainly had made lager beers before then. However, since fermentation was carried out by mixed yeast cultures and, without refrigeration, at relatively high temperatures, the "default" beer made by most of our forefathers had usually been an ale. The best lagers were made mostly during the winter months and then only in cooler regions, when and where nature was cooperative. Thanks to science and technology, by the end of the 19th century, man was able to brew both ales and lagers anywhere and of predictable quality.

Within a scant two decades from von Linde's invention of refrigeration, the conversion of German breweries from top fermentation to bottom fermentation was complete, except in the Rhineland. But even there, the commercial production of modern ale is plainly unthinkable without the use of pure, laboratory-managed, bacteria-free *saccharomyces cerevisiae* or without rigid temperature control of the mash and the fermenting wort.

Advances in technology, especially steam generation and refrigeration, also made brewing more capital-intensive and many small breweries folded or were taken over in Germany (and in the rest of the world) as industrialization with its large-scale factory breweries arrived in the 19th century. Breweries could expand their markets beyond the local horizon as the railway quickly replaced the horse-drawn dray for beer transport. In fact, the very first freight ever transported by a German railway were two casks of beer brewed by the Lederer Brewery of Nürnberg! The casks traveled to Fürth on July 11, 1836, on the first German rail link, a mere seven months after it had been opened.

While there are even today small local breweries and micro-breweries owned by nobles, convents, monasteries or private individuals, these do not account for a large share of the output of the German beer industry. Munich, for instance, boasted some 67 breweries in 1750. Within a century and a half, this number shrank to just a few large ones, such as Augustiner, Hacker-Pschorr, Löwenbräu, Paulaner-Salvator-Thomasbräu, Spaten-Franziskanerbräu, and Staatliches Hofbräuhaus. More than half the beer brewed in Bavaria now comes from a handful of these large corporations.

In Cologne, there were still about 120, mostly small, ale

breweries, in 1860. There were about 100 in Düsseldorf. By the end of the First World War, however, only about half of them remained in the two cities, and of those, fewer than half were small craft brewpubs. By the end of the Second World War, only 21 breweries survived in Cologne, incidentally the same number that started Cologne's Fraternity of Brewers in 1438. Today, the number of Kölsch breweries has rebounded slightly to 24. In Düsseldorf, 18 breweries survived the destruction of the Second World War. Of those, only two large ones and four brewpubs have weathered the mergers of the last few decades.

According to a Boston Globe report of October, 1996, there are about 1,200 breweries left in Germany, but their numbers are declining. More than 130 have closed between 1990 and 1995 alone. However, the Germans' love affair with beer is far from over. German breweries still produce a staggering 115 million hectoliters (almost 100 million barrels) a year and each German still drinks about 140 liters (about 37 gallons) of the stuff each year (statistical average for 1995). By comparison, Americans manage to down about 85 liters (22 gallons) a year.

Beer is still the anchor of popular culture in Germany. There is hardly a country in the world with so many drinking songs. And they are still being sung! Just visit a German pub during Mardigras, which is called Fasching in the south, Fassenacht in Hesse and Karneval in the north, and you can watch the otherwise so serious and reserved Germans loosen up over a mug of suds. In the beer halls of the land, it is quite customary for strangers to share long tables, to join arms and to sway in unison, from side to side, in a jovial sing-along. When entering a German pub or restaurant, you do not wait to be seated, as you would in North America. Germans are, perhaps surprisingly, social eaters and drinkers. While in North

America, restaurant patrons expect to be seated separately, every "party of one" or "party of two" with its own table that might actually seat four, Germans pick their own seating in restaurants, often preferring vacant seats at an already occupied table to the solitude of single dining.

Among the younger crowd, you may still encounter the custom of Stiefeltrinken ("boot drinking"). A glass boot, containing one or two liters of beer, makes the rounds at a large table, non-stop, from one occupant to another. Each drinker takes turns placing the tip of the boot in the air and taking a careful sip. As the beer level gets closer and closer to the boot's ankle, eventually, air would be sucked into the tip, displacing the beer that is there and splattering the drinker's face. The object of the game, however, is to avoid getting splashed by quickly twisting the tip of the boot downwards as soon as the air begins to rush in, without taking your mouth off the rim of the boot. Anybody who misses the moment and does get splashed, has to order (and pay for) the next boot. Obviously, those who are clever at this game, can imbibe with their friends all night without spending a penny.

Indeed, if you watch carefully, you can still detect in modern Germans, assembled in a pub or beer hall, a bit of the tribal frolicker that the Roman historian Tacitus described so well some 2,000 years ago.

3 Beer in the USA

Beer Brewing in The United States

Brewing in America dates to the first communities established by English and Dutch settlers in the early to mid-seventeenth century. Dutch immigrants quickly recognized that the climate and terrain of present-day New York were particularly well suited to brewing beer and growing malt and hops, two of beer's essential ingredients. A 1660 map of New Amsterdam details twenty-six breweries and taverns, a clear indication that producing and selling beer were popular and profitable trades in the American colonies. Despite the early popularity of beer, other alcoholic beverages steadily grew in importance and by the early eighteenth century several of them had eclipsed beer commercially.

Between 1650 and the Civil War, the market for beer did not change a great deal: both production and consumption remained essentially local affairs. Bottling was expensive, and beer did not travel well. Nearly all beer was stored in, and then served from, wooden kegs. While there were many small breweries, it was not uncommon for households to brew their own beer. In fact, several of America's founding fathers brewed their own beer, including George Washington and Thomas Jefferson.

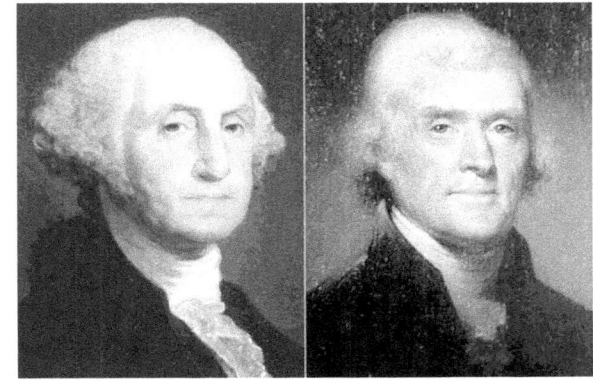

National production statistics are unavailable before 1810, an omission which reflects the rather limited importance of the early brewing industry. In 1810, America's 140 commercial breweries collectively produced just over 180,000 barrels of beer. During the next fifty years, total beer output continued to increase, but production remained small scale and local. This is not to suggest, however, that brewing could not prove profitable. In 1797, James Vassar founded a brewery in Poughkeepsie, New York whose successes echoed far beyond the brewing industry. After several booming years, Vassar ceded control of the brewery to his two sons, Matthew and John. Following the death of his brother in an accident and a fire that destroyed the plant, Matthew Vassar rebuilt the brewery in 1811. Demand for his beer grew rapidly, and by the early 1840s, the Vassar brewery produced nearly 15,000 barrels of ale and porter annually, a significant amount for this period. Continued investment in the firm facilitated even greater production levels, and by 1860 its fifty employees turned out 30,000 barrels of beer, placing it amongst the nation's largest breweries. Today, the Vassar name is better known for the college Matthew Vassar endowed in 1860 with earnings from the brewery.

While there were several hundred small scale, local breweries in the 1840s and 1850s, beer did not become a mass-produced, mass-consumed beverage until the decades following the Civil War. Several factors contributed to beer's emergence as the nation's dominant alcoholic drink.

- First, widespread immigration from strong beer drinking countries such as Britain, Ireland, and Germany contributed to the creation of a beer culture in the US.
- Second, America was becoming increasingly industrialized and urbanized during these years, and many workers in the

manufacturing and mining sectors drank beer during work and after.

- Third, many workers began to receive higher wages and salaries during these years, enabling them to buy more beer.
- Fourth, beer benefited from members of the temperance movement who advocated lower alcohol beer over higher alcohol spirits such as rum or whiskey.
- Fifth, a series of technological and scientific developments fostered greater beer production and the brewing of new styles of beer. For example, artificial refrigeration enabled brewers to brew during warm American summers, and pasteurization, the eponymous procedure developed by Louis Pasteur, helped extend packaged beer's shelf life, making storage and transportation more reliable (Stack, 2000).
- Finally sixth, American brewers began brewing lager beer, a style that had long been popular in Germany and other continental European countries. Traditionally, beer in America meant British-style ale. Ales are brewed with top fermenting yeasts, and this category ranges from light pale ales to chocolate-colored stouts and porters.

During the 1840s, American brewers began making German-style lager beers. In addition to requiring a longer maturation period than ales, lager beers use a bottom fermenting yeast and are much more temperature sensitive. Lagers require a great deal of care and attention from brewers, but to the increasing numbers of nineteenth century German immigrants, lager was synonymous with beer. As the nineteenth century wore on, lager production soared, and by 1900, lager outsold ale by a significant margin.

Together, these factors helped transform the market for beer. Total beer production increased from 3.6 million barrels in 1865 to over 66 million barrels in 1914. By 1910, brewing had grown into one of the leading manufacturing industries in America. Yet, this increase in output did not simply reflect America's growing

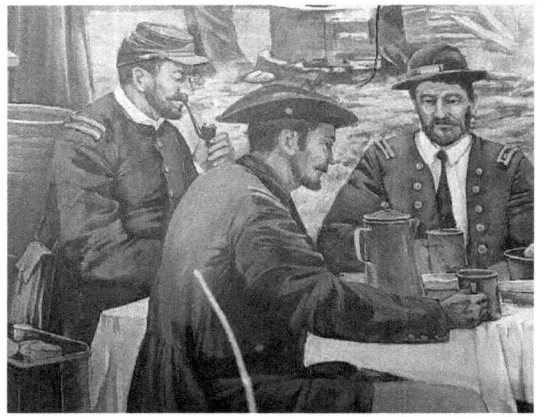

population. While the number of beer drinkers certainly did rise during these years, perhaps just as importantly, per capita consumption also rose dramatically, from under four gallons in 1865 to 21 gallons in the early 1910s.

An equally impressive transformation was underway at the level of the firm. Until the 1870s and 1880s, American breweries had been essentially small scale, local operations. By the late nineteenth century, several companies began to increase their scale of production and scope of distribution. Pabst Brewing Company in Milwaukee and Anheuser-Busch in St. Louis became two of the nation's first nationally-oriented breweries, and the first to surpass annual production levels of one million barrels. By utilizing the growing railroad system to distribute significant amounts of their beer into distant beer markets, Pabst, Anheuser-Busch and a handful of other enterprises came to be called "shipping" breweries. Though these firms became very powerful, they did not control the pre-Prohibition market for beer. Rather, an equilibrium emerged that pitted large and regional shipping breweries that incorporated the latest innovations in pasteurizing, bottling, and transporting beer against a great number of locally-oriented breweries that mainly supplied draught beer in wooden kegs to their immediate markets.

Between the Civil War and national prohibition, the production and consumption of beer greatly outpaced spirits. Though consumption levels of absolute alcohol had peaked in the early 1800s, temperance and prohibition forces grew increasingly vocal and active as the century wore on, and by the late 1800s, they constituted one of the best-organized political pressure groups of the day. Their efforts culminated in the ratification of the Eighteenth Amendment on January 29, 1919 that, along with the Volstead Act, made the production and distribution of any beverages with more than one-half of one percent alcohol illegal. While estimates of alcohol activity during Prohibition's thirteen-year reign, from 1920 to 1933, are imprecise, beer consumption almost certainly fell, though spirit consumption may have remained constant or actually even increased slightly.

The most important decision all breweries had to make after 1920 was what to do with their plants and equipment. As they grappled with this question, they made implicit bets as to whether Prohibition would prove to be merely a temporary irritant. Pessimists immediately divested themselves of all their brewing equipment, often at substantial losses. Other firms decided to carry

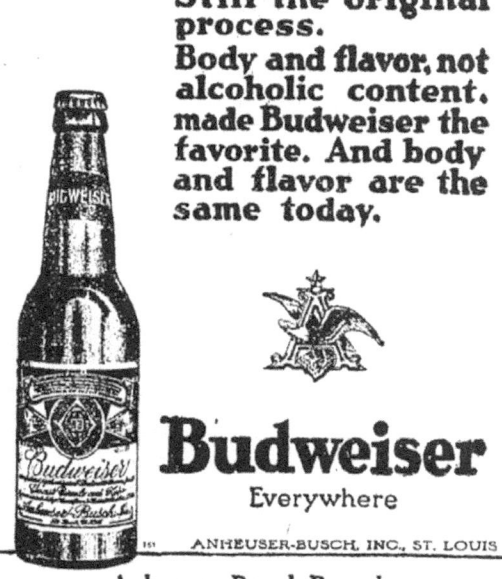

Still the original process.
Body and flavor, not alcoholic content, made Budweiser the favorite. And body and flavor are the same today.

Budweiser
Everywhere

ANHEUSER-BUSCH, INC., ST. LOUIS

Anheuser-Busch Branch
Wholesale Distributors
Washington, District of Columbia

on with related products, and so stay prepared for any modifications to the Volstead Act which would allow for beer. Schlitz, Blatz, Pabst, and Anheuser-Busch, the leading pre-Prohibition shippers, began producing near beer, a malt beverage with under one-half of one percent alcohol. While it was not a commercial success, its production allowed these firms to keep current their beer-making skills. Anheuser-Busch called its near beer "Budweiser" which was "simply the old Budweiser lager beer, brewed according to the traditional method, and then de-alcoholized. Just check out the ad above.

August Busch took the same care in purchasing the costly materials as he had done during pre-prohibition days." Anheuser-Busch and some of the other leading breweries were granted special licenses by the federal government for brewing alcohol greater than one half of one percent for "medicinal purposes." Receiving these licensees gave these breweries a competitive advantage as they were able to keep their brewing staff active in beer-making.

The shippers, and some local breweries, also made malt syrup. While they officially advertised it as an ingredient for baking cookies, and while its production was left alone by the government, it was readily apparent to all that its primary use was for homemade beer.

Of perhaps equal importance to the day-to-day business activities of the breweries were their investment decisions. Here, as in so many other places, the shippers exhibited true entrepreneurial insight. Blatz, Pabst, and Anheuser-Busch all expanded their inventories of automobiles and trucks, which became key assets after repeal. In the 1910s, Anheuser-Busch invested in motorized vehicles to deliver beer; by the 1920s, it was building its own trucks in great numbers. While it never sought to become a major producer of delivery vehicles, its forward expansion in this area reflected its appreciation of the growing importance of motorized delivery, an insight which they built on after repeal.

The leading shippers also furthered their investments in bottling equipment and machinery, which was used in the production of near beer, root beer, ginger ale, and soft drinks. These products were not the commercial successes beer had been, but they gave breweries important experience in bottling. While 85 percent of pre-Prohibition beer was kegged, during Prohibition over 80 percent of near beer and a smaller, though growing, percentage of soft drinks was sold in bottles.

This remarkable increase in packaged product impelled breweries to refine their packaging skills and modify their retailing practice. As they sold near beer and soft drinks to drugstores and drink stands, they encountered new marketing problems. Experience gained during these years helped the shippers meet radically different distribution requirements of the post-repeal beer market.

They were learning about canning as well as bottling. In 1925, Blatz's canned malt syrup sales were more than $1.3 million, significantly greater than its bulk sales. Anheuser-Busch used cans from the American Can Company for its malt syrup in the early 1920s, a firm which would gain national prominence in 1935 for helping to pioneer the beer can. Thus, the canning of malt syrup helped create the first contacts between the leading shipping brewers and American Can Company. These expensive investments in automobiles and bottling equipment were paid for in part by selling off branch properties, namely saloons. Some had equipped their saloons with furniture and bar fixtures, but as Prohibition wore on, they progressively divested themselves of these assets.

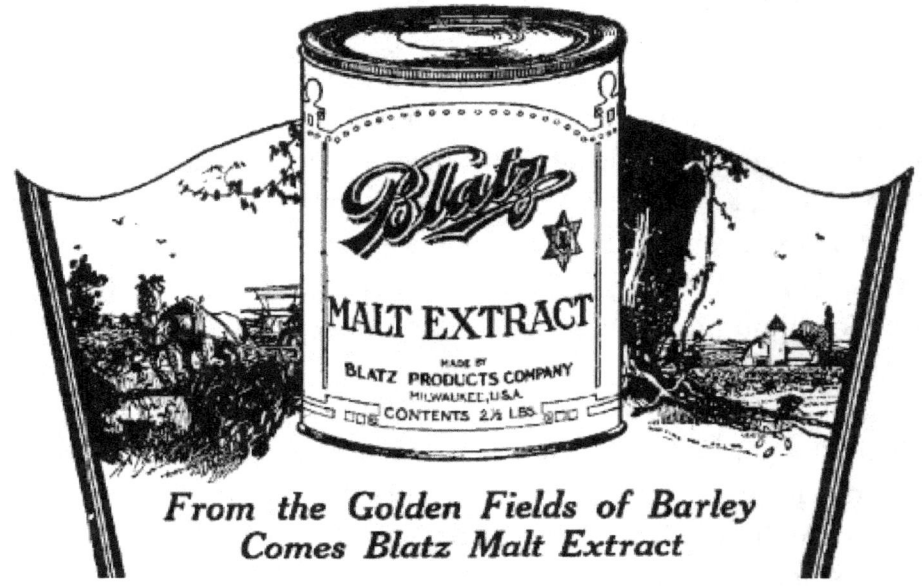

**From the Golden Fields of Barley
Comes Blatz Malt Extract**

In April 1933 Congress amended the Volstead Act to allow for 3.2 percent beer. Eight months later, in December, Congress and the states ratified the Twenty-first Amendment, officially repealing Prohibition. From repeal until World War II, the brewing industry struggled to regain its pre-Prohibition fortunes. Prior to prohibition, breweries owned or controlled many saloons, which were the dominant retail outlets for alcohol. To prevent the excesses that had been attributed to saloons from reoccurring, post-repeal legislation forbade alcohol manufacturers from owning bars or saloons, requiring them instead to sell their beer to wholesalers that in turn would distribute their beverages to retailers.

Prohibition meant the end of many small breweries that had been profitable, and that, taken together, had posed a formidable challenge to the large shipping breweries. The shippers, who had

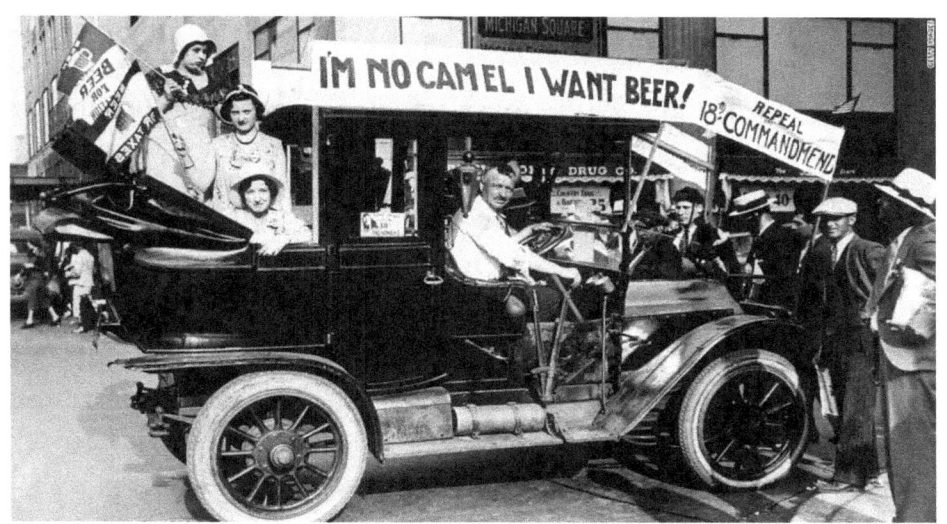

much greater investments, were not as inclined to walk away from brewing. After repeal, therefore, they reopened for business in a radically new environment, one in which their former rivals were absent or disadvantaged. From this favorable starting point, they continued to consolidate their position. Several hundred locally oriented breweries did reopen, but were unable to regain their pre-Prohibition competitive edge, and they quickly exited the market. From 1935 to 1940, the number of breweries fell by ten percent.

Annual industry output, after struggling in 1934 and 1935, began to approach the levels reached in the 1910s. Yet, these total increases are somewhat misleading, as the population of the U.S. had risen from 92 to 98 million in the 1910s to 125 to 130 million in the 1930s. This translated directly into lower per capita consumption levels during this time. The largest firms grew even larger in the years following repeal, quickly surpassing their pre-Prohibition annual production levels. The post-repeal industry leaders, Anheuser-Busch and Pabst, doubled their annual levels of production from 1935 to 1940.

To take for granted the growing importance of the leading shippers during this period is to ignore their momentous reversal of pre-Prohibition trends. While medium-sized breweries dominated the industry output in the years leading up to Prohibition, the shippers regained in the 1930s the dynamism they manifested from the 1870s to the 1890s. From 1877 to 1895, Anheuser-Busch and Pabst, the two most prominent shippers, grew much faster than the industry, and their successes helped pull the industry along. This picture changed during the years 1895 to 1915, when the *industry* grew much faster than the shippers. With the repeal of Prohibition, the tides changed yet again: from 1934 to 1940, the brewing industry grew very slowly, while Anheuser-Busch and Pabst enjoyed tremendous increases in their annual sales.

National and regional shippers increasingly dominated the market. Breweries such as Anheuser-Busch, Pabst and Schlitz came to exemplify the modern business enterprise, as described by Alfred Chandler, which adeptly integrated mass production and mass distribution.

World War One had presented a direct threat to the brewing industry. Government officials used war-time emergencies to impose grain rationing, a step that led to the lowering of the alcohol level of beer to 2.75 percent. World War Two had a completely different effect on the industry: rather than output falling, beer production rose from 1941 to 1945. During the Second World War, the industry mirrored the nation at large by casting off its sluggish depression-era growth. As the war economy boomed, consumers, both troops and civilians, used some of their wages for beer, and per capita consumption grew by 50 percent between 1940 and 1945. Yet, the take-off registered during the World War II was not sustained during the ensuing decades. Total production continued to grow, but at a slower rate than overall population. Beer was looked at very differently in the Second World War, it was seen as a war necessity!

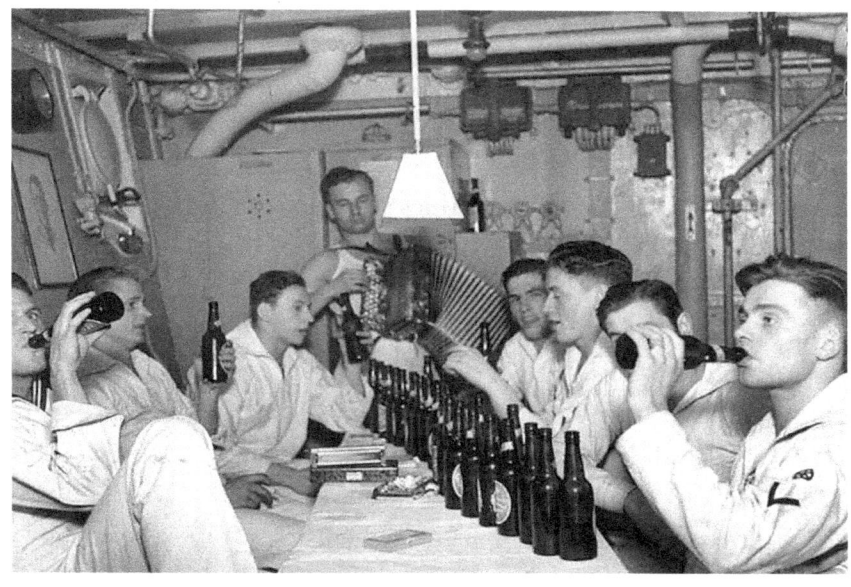

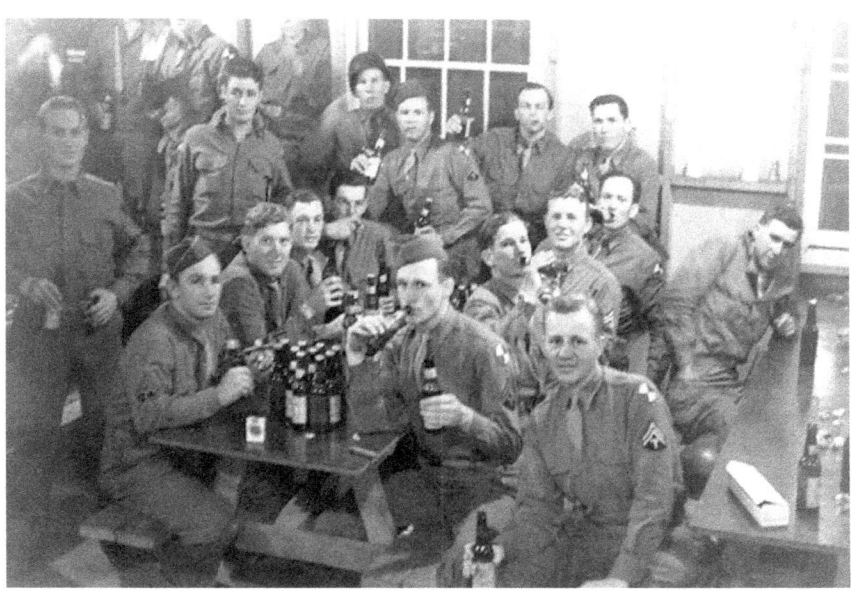

No one would ever argue with the reality that war is tough, and that the men and women who elect to serve are a truly special breed. But it might come as some surprise that during World War II the British and US governments believed soldiers were so vital that they were willing to go to great lengths in order to supply them with a substance they felt was incredibly important for their morale: **beer!**

The problem was that for soldiers stationed in the Pacific, the beer was pretty terrible. This was true for two main reasons: the first was that our British and American beers didn't travel all that well, meaning that by the time they finally arrived at the base, they were pretty skunked and often tasted quite rancid. The second reason was that there weren't many local options. The country we were fighting, Japan, wasn't really making beer, and as for sake, the Japanese had either converted those breweries into munitions factories, or were giving what was left to their Kamikaze pilots.

But we didn't want to leave our soldiers in the lurch, drinking only skunky beer in an attempt to raise their spirits, so what did we do? Drop it by aircraft? Nope. (Well, we actually tried it but it did not deliver enough beer – the containers tended to burst open on impact.)

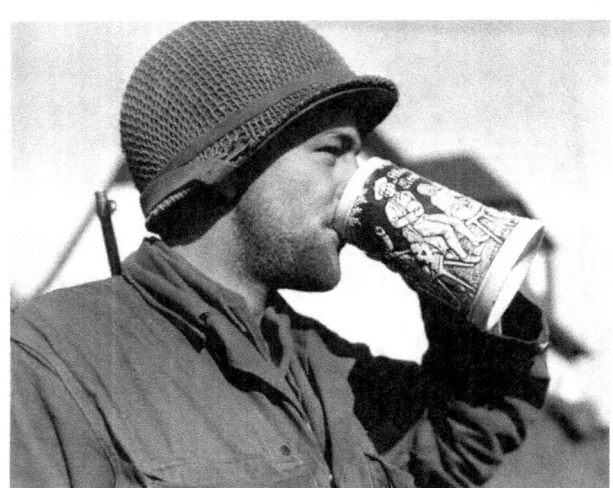

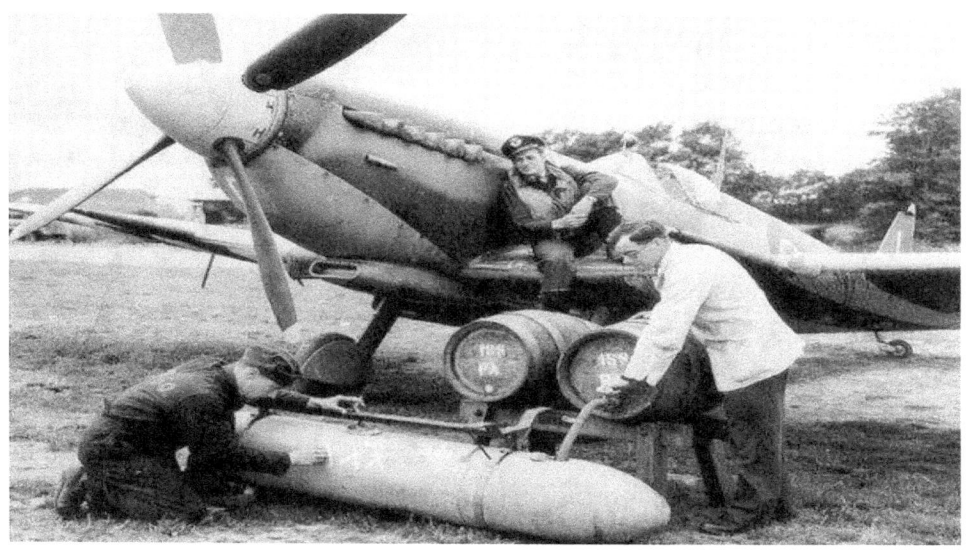

We built brewery ships! Well, OK — the British actually built the brewery ships, but since we're allies, they were willing to share. These ships were built at the insistence of Winston Churchill himself and were not only to include breweries, but also cinemas, dance halls and other amenities, which is why they then became known as amenity ships.

The original plan was for the British Navy to build ten of these ships and station them across the Pacific, allowing them to supply allied troops with all the sudsy sustenance they desired. To build these floating breweries, the British converted old mine-laying ships, outfitting the hulls with a 55-barrel capacity brewing pot. The brewing pot was heated with steam coils powered by the ship's boiler, and six glass lined fermenting vessels, capable of churning out 250 barrels of beer per week. In the end however, only two of these ships came to fruition, as the war ended before production was even able to begin on the other eight.

These two ships, the HMS Menestheus and the Agamemnon were built in Western Canada, though the Agamemnon never wound up leaving the shipping yard. Only the HMS Menestheus set sail from Canada for the Pacific towards the end of the war, with the ship's

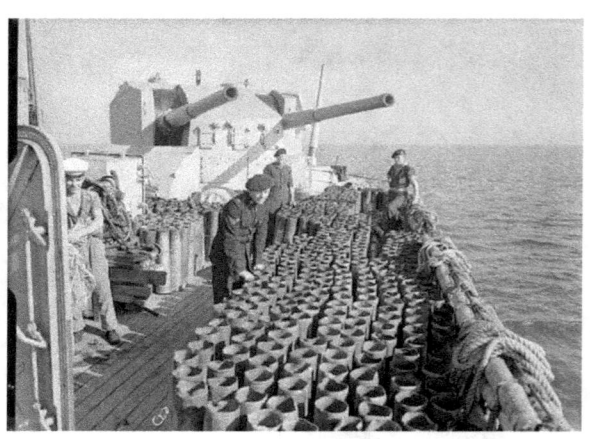

first batch of beer brewed on the last day of 1945.

Although the war was over shortly after the HMS Menestheus's arrival, allied troops still remained and the beer they were drinking was still terrible, so the ship began its critical role of supplying those troops with palatable beer. During its time in the Pacific the HMS Menestheus visited the ports of Yokohama, Kure, Shanghai and Hong Kong, brewing a mild ale that was served slightly chilled.

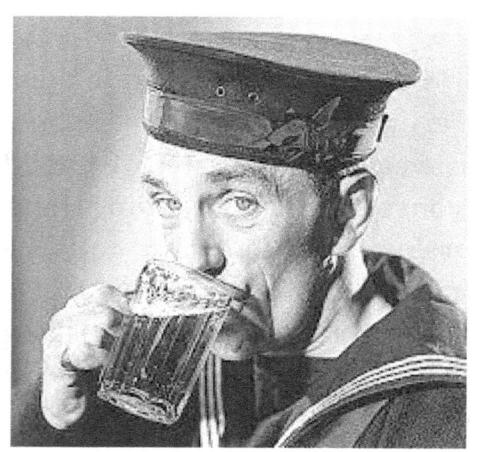

Reports from soldiers who consumed it at the time were that the beer was absolutely delicious, especially when compared to what they had been drinking before. Who knows, had the brewery ships come to fruition earlier in the campaign, both sides might have decided to simply work out their differences over a delicious pint!

The period following WWII was characterized by great industry consolidation. Total output continued to grow, though per capita consumption fell into the 1960s before rebounding to levels above 21 gallons per capita in the 1970s, the highest rates in the nation's history. Not since the 1910s, had consumption levels topped 21 gallons a year; however, there was a significant difference. Prior to Prohibition most consumers bought their beer from local or regional firms and over 85 percent of the beer was served from casks in saloons. Following World War II, two significant changes radically altered the market for beer. First, the total number of breweries operating fell dramatically. This signaled the growing importance of the large national breweries. While many of these firms — Anheuser-Busch, Pabst, Schlitz, and Blatz — had grown into prominence in the late nineteenth century, the scale of their operations grew tremendously in the years after the repeal of prohibition. From the mid- 1940s to 1980, the five largest breweries saw their share of the national market grow from 19 to 75 percent. The other important change concerned how beer was sold. Prior to Prohibition, nearly all beer was sold on-tap in bars or saloons; while approximately 10-15 percent of the beer was bottled, it was much more expensive than draught beer. In 1935, a few years after repeal, the American Can Company successfully canned beer for the first time. The spread of home refrigeration helped spur consumer demand for canned and bottled beer, and from 1935 onwards, draught beer sales have fallen markedly.

From 1980 to 2000, beer production continued to rise, reaching nearly 200 million barrels in 2000. Per capita consumption hit its highest recorded level in 1981 with 23.8 gallons. Since then, though, consumption levels have dropped a bit, and during the 1990s, consumption was typically in the 21-22 gallon range.

Beginning around 1980, the long decline in the number of

breweries slowed and then was reversed. Judging solely by the number of breweries in operation, it appeared that a significant change had occurred: the number of firms began to increase, and by the late 1990s, hundreds of new breweries were operating in the U.S. However, this number is rather misleading: the overall industry remained very concentrated, with a three-firm concentration ratio in 2000 of 81 percent.

Although entrepreneurs and beer enthusiasts began hundreds of new breweries during this period, most of them were very small, with annual production levels of between 5,000 to 100,000 barrels annually. Reflecting their small size, these new firms were called microbreweries. Collectively, microbreweries have grown to account for approximately 5-7 percent of the total beer market.

Microbreweries represented a new strategy in the brewing industry: rather than competing on the basis of price or advertising, they attempted to compete on the basis of inherent product characteristics. They emphasized the freshness of locally produced beer; they experimented with much stronger malt and hop flavors; they tried new and long-discarded brewing recipes, often reintroducing styles that had been popular in America decades earlier. Together, these breweries have had an influence much greater than their market share would suggest. The big three breweries, Anheuser Busch, Miller, and Coors, have all tried to incorporate ideas from the microbrewery movement. They have introduced new marquee brands intended to compete for some of this market, and when this failed, they have bought shares in or outright control of some microbreweries.

A final dimension of the brewing industry that has been changing concerns the emerging global market for beer. Until very recently, America was the biggest beer market in the world: as a result, American breweries have not historically looked abroad for additional sales, preferring to expand their share of the domestic market. In the1980s, Anheuser-Busch began to systematically evaluate its market position. While it had done very well in the US, it had not tapped markets overseas; as a result, it began a series of international business dealings. It gradually moved from exporting small amounts of its flagship brand Budwesier to entering into licensing accords whereby breweries in a range of countries such as Ireland, Japan, and Argentina began to brew Budweiser for sale in their domestic markets. In 1995, it established its first breweries outside of the US, one in England for the European market and the other in China, to service the growing markets in China and East Asia.

While US breweries such as Anheuser-Busch have only recently begun to explore the opportunities abroad, foreign firms have long appreciated the significance of the American market. Beginning in the late 1990s, imports began to increase their market share and by the early 2000s, they accounted for approximately 12 percent of the large U.S. market. Imports and microbrews typically cost more than the big three's beers and they provide a wider range of flavors and tastes. One of the most interesting developments in the international market for beer occurred in 2002 when South African Breweries (SAB), the dominant brewery in South Africa, and an active firm in Europe, acquired Miller, the second largest brewery in the US. Though not widely discussed in the US, this may portend a general move towards increased global integration in the world market for beer.

4. Food & Drink as Medicine!

"Let food be thy medicine and medicine be thy food." This quote is attributed to Hippocrates. Another of my favorite quotes is *"Who said anything about medicine? Let's eat!"* which is attributed to one of Hippocrates forgotten (and hilarious) students. The same can be said for the drinks we consume – like coffee.

Who hasn't seen or heard Hippocrates' famous quote above? If you have Facebook friends who are the least bit into "natural" medicine or living, you've almost certainly come across it in your feed, and if you're a reader of my Phytonutrient Blog, you will absolutely have heard the quote. Now Hippocrates lived a very long time ago, that is definitely true but just because an idea is old, doesn't mean it's good, any more than just because Hippocrates said it means it must be true. But in this case, it does and it is!

Remember, Hippocrates was an important figure in the history of medicine because he was among the earliest to assert that diseases were caused by natural processes rather than the gods and because of his emphasis on the careful observation and documentation of patient history and physical findings, which led to the discovery of physical signs associated with diseases of specific organs. He is also known to have been a great healer because of his knowledge of the culinary and medicinal uses of herbs and spices. But you know what? Hippocrates was not the only advocate for letting food be thy medicine. Throughout the ages there have been many others. Ever since man first climbed down from the trees (or, depending upon your view, plucked that apple off that tree), eating has never been far from his

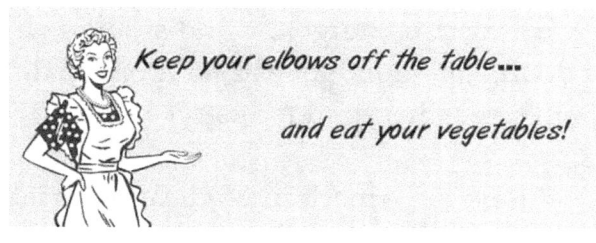

Keep your elbows off the table...

and eat your vegetables!

mind (survival has a way of prioritizing everything). The simple fact that sustenance equals life, means that food and health have culturally ridden shotgun throughout the ages.

"Good men eat and drink so they can live," noted Socrates.
"Eat, drink, and be merry!" commanded Solomon.
"You're famished. I'll fix you a plate!!" pleaded my mother.

In the days before medicine, food and drink was medicine...or at least it was seen as such. A browned apple for an upset stomach, chicken soup for congestion, champagne for septicemia (Pulitzer Prize-winning novelist Eudora Welty said her Mississippi father swore his use of the bubbly saved her ill mother's life). It was sometimes hard to establish cause and effect (Garlic as an anti-vampiric? Hard to find test subjects for that one,) and yet generations of pantries held foods sworn to bind, purge, ameliorate, instigate, invigorate...in short, improve one's well-being. And then came modern allopathic-oriented science, which until recently tossed nutrition—and its potential effect on both maintaining health and calming illness—into the compost heap. The reasons were myriad. Politically, no one had ever been elected on an anti-cheeseburger platform, so administrative pressure to funnel government dollars toward nutritional research traditionally was nil. Similarly, big pharma was scarce with cash, because they can't patent a food's natural properties. And from a practical viewpoint, studying food with its thousands of chemicals and nutrients is incredibly complex.

By comparison, targeting and studying a single drug for efficacy in a double-blind model was far more straightforward and lucrative to both researchers and industry.

It took the American Medical Association until 2002 to reverse a long-standing position and suggest that adults take a multivitamin every day. Then again, many of its long-standing members had never been exposed to a nutrition elective while in medical school...creating a drug-oriented bias that historically expressed itself in both the clinic and the lab.

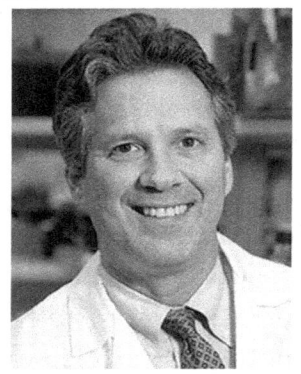

"I think for a long time the major directions in molecular biology—the ability to make genetically altered mice that could measure the impacts of certain molecules on the body—was totally not applied to nutrition," - Hopkins' William Nelson, director of the Sidney Kimmel Cancer Center.

That Nelson can speak of such research deficiencies in the past tense is indicative of a huge shift toward nutritional research in just the past 10 to 15 years. Again, I remind you that the information I present in this series, while in truth very old is now being backed by 21st Century science and research!

What then is the catalyst for this paradigm shift in thinking? Well since you asked I'll tell you what I think. We can't seem to shut our mouths, and the stats from the Centers for Disease Control back that up! With the exception of Colorado dwellers, more than 20% of the U.S. population is now considered obese. Given obesity's epidemiologically supported impact on cardiac, vascular, cancer, and diabetic-related illness, researchers are now branching out to uncover the myriad ways food and its micro components enhance or disrupt life. The sheer numbers of nutritional studies bear out this interest. According to Pub Med, such published investigations more than doubled between the 1980s and 1990s, and leapt another 71% this decade. Part of the quantum leap in the last five years especially, is the discovery that chronic inflammation is slowly being linked to diseases including cancer, and that foods—from cloves to walnuts—appear to contain anti-inflammatory properties.

This critical mass of information even has a name. Called the 'Food as Medicine movement', it's a growing recognition on the part of many academic clinicians that to ignore the role of food and nutrition in health is to lose a valuable tool that can support (or perhaps even lessen or replace) many pharmaceuticals currently in use.

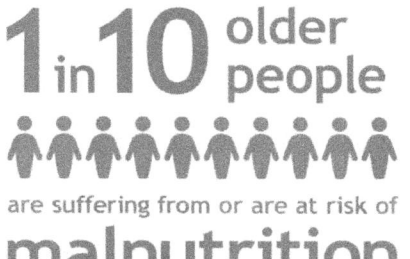

1 in 10 older people

are suffering from or are at risk of

malnutrition *"The perfect example is ginger,"* says Hopkins gastroenterologist Gerard Mullin, arguably the nation's top expert on the relationship between food and gut disorders. *"People who have nausea, or gastric dysmotilities or other GI problems, for them ginger is at the top of my list. It works the same way (the big pharma produced) Zofran does, which is one of our most powerful anti-nausea drugs. It works on the same receptor in the brain. But many docs aren't aware of it."*

Similarly, food plays a huge role in how well people battle cancer. Researchers estimate that some 80% of cancer patients are malnourished, at the very time when chemotherapy often increases the body's need for proteins and other nutrients. Such malnourishment, if not addressed, can lead to a reduction of chemotherapy doses and ultimately poorer outcomes. Oncologist Bill Nelson says that the link between calories taken in—the so-called "caloric budget"—and its relationship to cancer is of great interest to him. Nelson notes that caloric intake drops among the elderly, while their cancer rates rise. It may well be that taking in fewer calories—especially of food of little to no nutritional value—leaves elders deprived of nutrients they need to stave off cancer, he says.

The thirst for nutritional knowledge is by no means limited to physicians and wellness professionals. A poll of attendees of <u>A Women's Journey</u>, an annual women's health symposium sponsored by Hopkins Medicine, showed a huge demand for more seminars devoted to the nuances of nutrition, and faculty speakers who could make sense of the flood of dietary data being unleashed on the public. In response, the Fall 2009 <u>A Woman's Journey</u> featured numerous talks with a nutritional component, including three seminars—led by the aforementioned Nelson, Mullin, and nutritionist Lynda McIntyre—that, like a well-balanced meal, triangulated how different research approaches are translating into smarter ways to eat for health. For Gerard Mullin, nutrition and health have always been intertwined. What's different now is the scientific rigor being applied to the field.

"My mom had the first health food store in northern New Jersey. I've cooked since I was 10," says Mullin. *"I was raised on food as medicine, and I'm glad the science has really borne out and supported what many of us were raised to believe since we were yay high."* Mullin refers to himself as an integrative gastroenterologist, the adjective referring to physicians who use complementary modalities including stress management and nutrition in their clinical practices. In both interviews and talks, Mullin lays out a compelling explanation for the mind/body connection to the gut, and

how different foods, spices, and herbs can promote better digestive health, especially in the 90 million Americans suffering from digestive diseases. He focuses on the common negative feedback loop affecting the "cephalic" phase of digestion—the gastric and saliva secretions that occur when appetite is stimulated but before eating actually begins. Sleep deprivation, emotional upset, poor eating habits—all can lead to an impaired cephalic phase. It's the stomach's equivalent of not being in the mood, and the response is somewhat the same. Diminished blood flow impairs function: In this case the gut doesn't absorb nutrients. All that unabsorbed food can make us miserable (i.e., everything from diarrhea to gas, bloating, and beyond). That jacks up stress levels, makes eating even more undesirable, and before you know it you've worked yourself into a case of irritable bowel syndrome or worse.

While drugs can treat symptoms, Mullin says breaking the cycle is both a mental and physical process. Taking the time to cook can in itself enhance that first cephalic phase—everything from the meditative act of chopping to inhaling rich aromas can be relaxing— while choosing certain foods such as peppermint leaves and ground flax may reduce gut spasms.

According to British Medical Journal studies, Mullin says, *"Peppermint works better than most IBS drugs. It works on relaxing calcium channel blockers.*

1 in 3 people aged 65+

are at risk of malnutrition

on admission to hospital

Sometimes it can make your gut so relaxed, right between the gut and esophagus, that you get some burping or heartburn, so you have to be careful how much you use. More isn't always better."

At Hopkins, Mullin has worked to improve both nutrition and timely access to food given to Johns Hopkins Hospital inpatients. *"In a hospital setting, anywhere from 33% to 55% of people are malnourished,"* he notes. With study funding from Department of Medicine Chief Mike Weisfeldt, says Mullin, "we proved that if you feed people earlier (following admission), their hospital stay is shorter and outcome is much better. It is common sense, but we had to show the evidence. And it's reawakened a whole discussion" about improving gut health through diet. Mullin notes that many common kitchen staples can be very effective for preventing and relieving gut-related maladies. *"Caraway has been well-studied,"* Mullin says. *"Its oil is a treatment for gastroparesis, so for those with slow motility and problems with their upper GI tract, caraway can promote motility. Fennel, ginger, dill, cumin...all these things can help you on an everyday basis."*

From both a taste and nutrient viewpoint, fresh is generally better than dried, though dried is better than nothing. As for amounts, most research suggests moderation as a key, the idea being that it's the continuous, sustainable addition of herbs and other nutrients that enhance flavor and long-term gut health. Do not skip meals, eating regularly and including herbs and spices, fruit and vegetables, and fish is truly necessary to optimum health especially in our young and elderly.

Equally important is what foods to avoid. Improving that cephalic response will be pretty much a waste if the gut is being overdosed with junk. Mullin cites studies noting that, while the average American consumes 100 grams of fructose a day—

22% of people aged 60+ **skipped meals** to cut back on **food costs**

everything from "soda to ketchup to grapes"—the body can only tolerate about 50 grams. The overload acts as an IBS and gas trigger. *"The first thing we do is say, 'Look, if you want to get better, you have to find a way to eliminate some of these sugars."* He says. Mullin aims his last culinary salvo at inflammation. Many scientists believe that certain aspects of lifestyle—notably what we eat—can create a chronic inflammatory state within cells, tissues, and organs. In short, the immune system is in constant attack mode, which may have deleterious effects on health. *"We know that many conditions in the gut are mediated through inflammation. We're appreciating that now more than ever,"* he says, pointing to recent research links. *"How do you help make yourself better? Again, it's a food as medicine approach. There are (anti-inflammatory) studies about blueberries and blackberries out there (see "Allies in the Pantry.")*

Bill Nelson's interest in food literally comes down to a flip of the wrist. No, not as a chef, but rather a scientist fascinated by how foods—notably meats—are altered by the way they're cooked. Using World Health Organization data, Nelson concluded that some 35% of cancers probably include a dietary element, with inflammation—which could also have dietary factors—playing a role in perhaps another 30% of cases. A highly respected molecular biologist and cancer clinician—he's principal investigator for one of the National Cancer Institute's Specialized Program of Research Excellence (SPORE) initiatives—Nelson has taken a microscopic interest in the interplay of diet and prostate cancer. He notes that not only do Asian men have far less prostate cancer than their American counterparts, they appear far less prone to inflammation. When comparing autopsies of non-cancerous prostates of men who live in America versus those in Asia, *"Every prostate removed here showed signs of inflammation, while the Asian prostates were pristine."* Curiously, the longer Asian men are in America, the more likely they are to develop prostate cancer. *"If they're here 25 years or more, their rate becomes half that of Caucasians, and if their kids are born here, their risk is the same as Caucasians. There must be something in the lifestyle risks that we can reduce."* While Asians tend to eat far more fish and far less meat and fowl than Americans, Nelson says that might not tell the whole story. The problem may lie in how we heat our meats. *"Heat changes a huge amount of the components in food,"* says Nelson, focusing on two particular carcinogens that can be created by cooking. The first, called heterocyclic amines, are formed by the heat-catalyzed interplay between creatinine (found in the muscle of meats and fish) and amino acids.

One heterocyclic amine called "PhIP" is extremely nasty: When given to rats in doses comparable to those consumed by humans, the male rats rapidly developed prostate and colon cancer, while the female rats developed colon and breast cancer.

"For us, that was fascinating," recalled Nelson. *"We just said, 'Holy cow! It is incredible that something you could eat could do that."*

37% 🏠
of people aged
70+ who have recently moved into care homes are at risk of
malnutrition

Not only can the amount and duration of heat increase these dangerous amines (i.e., well-done appears worse for you than medium or medium rare), but so can cooking technique. *"You can take burger patties, put them on the same skillet, control for temperature and time, but in one case you flip them only once, in the middle of cooking, while the other you flip every 30 seconds."* The burgers only flipped once *"make a ton of amines,"* notes Nelson. *"So did sausages cooked as links versus patties."* The links, in Nelson's opinion, act *"as closed reaction vessels."* Nelson's own research uncovered that in many cases the liver can't metabolize all these "charred" meat carcinogens, and passes them through to the prostate, where people with a particular DNA mutation may be at much higher risk for developing cancer.

Nelson also points out that the fat dripping along a deep grilled steak might taste delicious, but it's potentially deadly. The culprit, which also escapes from the fat in chicken skin, is something called polycyclic aromatic hydrocarbon carcinogens. To put some numbers to the science, Nelson says the amount of these carcinogens consumed daily by the average American *"equals ingesting half a pack of cigarette smoke a day."*

My suggestion: **If you're going to eat meat, and I am, then stick to lower-fat cuts, take the skin off of chicken before cooking, and look at alternatives such as broiling or, in the case of fish, poaching the filet. Remember too that fat in the diet is important, but it is the right fats – like olive oil or the fats that are found in fish that we need – not a ton of beef or poultry fats.**

Nelson believes that both the public and industry are ready to hear his message. In meetings with executives at a large grocery store, Nelson discovered that 16% of the chain's sales came from pre-cooked foods and meals that busy customers quickly reheated at home. The executives had quite an appetite for Nelson's food prep science. Not only would such techniques improve food safety, but long term, the executives saw such preparatory expertise as potentially marketable to health-conscious consumers. *"I'm tantalized by the way we could affect broad-based cooking practices,"* he says *"We're at the dawn of an era of figuring this out."*

Figuring out how to translate serious science into tasty, healthy snacks and meals is where nutritionist Lynda McIntyre excels. A registered dietitian with a specialty counseling cancer patients at both the Kimmel Cancer Center at Hopkins and the Sibley Hospital Center for Breast Health in Washington D.C., McIntyre took A Woman's Journey attendees on a virtual tour of the supermarket.

Along the way, she busted some myths regarding what it is about food that links it to perhaps the majority of cancer cases.

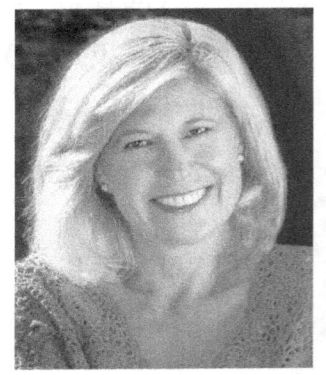

"A lot of times people think I'm talking about pesticides or additives in food, when in fact I'm not," she says. *"Less than 2% percent of all cancers can be directly related to what the additives are in food. Up to 60 percent can be related to what we're not eating."*

Read that quote again – I know that we are all concerned about pesticides in our food, as we should be, but we need to be at least equally concerned about what **we are and are not eating!** As in enough fruits and vegetables. A familiar message, yes, but McIntyre gives it a twist, suggesting shoppers take a colorful approach to solving their qualms about which produce has the greatest overall benefits. You have heard me say it and now this doctor stresses it too, *"Eat the rainbow. The brighter the food, the richer the color, the higher its anti-oxidant count,"* counsels McIntyre, who also served on a statewide council that developed cancer prevention strategies for Maryland. For McIntyre and other savvy nutritionists, the state of food science has allowed them to fine-tune their message and take some of the confusion out of the game. Take fresh versus frozen produce. McIntyre says both are effective…

"Fresh is always best when it is in season," says McIntyre, since fresh produce retains top flavor and nutritional value. However, McIntyre notes that many fresh foods have relatively short seasons. As an alternative, from a nutritional viewpoint, *"frozen can be just as nutritious because it's picked at the peak of ripeness, and frozen to keep the nutritional content intact."*

Then there's eating whole foods versus taking supplements, a source of huge debate. The prevailing sentiment among many researchers is that supplementation can bring someone deficient in a given nutrient up to a supportive baseline, but people already at solid baseline levels may not benefit from additional dosing.

93% of malnourished older people are in the **community.**

"In some cases, single supplementation of antioxidants can increase the risk of certain diseases," says McIntyre. *"For example, vitamin E and heart disease. Another example is that single supplementation of vitamin A can increase bone fractures in women. And in smokers who took beta-carotene, we saw an increase in lung cancer. The studies show it is the whole foods (and how they work together synergistically) that provides the most protective effect to the body."*

Knowing how to combine those foods can increase the body's ability to absorb their nutrients. McIntyre says putting broccoli (sulforaphane) and tomatoes (lycopene) together *"increases their tumor protective ability."* Similarly, carrots and avocado are a nice dynamic duo because beta-carotene is better absorbed in the presence of a fat (short on avocados? Try olive oil). Apples and blueberries, even spinach and strawberries (*"It's a strange combination, but delicious,"* insists McIntyre) all make for nutrient-dense dynamic duos.

Now for the bottom line, what I want, and need, for you to understand is this; as for the thinking that healthy eating and drinking is restrictive, forget it. Nearly every family of food and beverage that I have researched—be it nut, fruit, spice, fish, grain, beans, chocolate, wine, beer or coffee, has some and very often many, members in it filled with high nutritional content, when we consume them in moderation. On every conceivable front, from the molecular level to the kitchen table, research is unlocking the power of certain foods and drinks to keep us in fighting shape. Since none of us has a "foodprint" yet—a DNA or some other molecular roadmap that will tell us why Sally's system can absorb beta-carotene from carrots, while Sue's can only assimilate that same beta-carotene from sweet potatoes—for now, eating a well-rounded, well-informed diet containing moderate amounts of a wide varieties of fresh foods and drinks, is all about playing the odds. And there's nothing better than improving your chances of beating the house.

So, the next time that someone tries to tell you that you shouldn't be drinking that Miller Lite – just tell them that they shouldn't worry, you are just working on improving your health!

5 Health Benefits of Beer

Sure, you probably have beer to thank for helping you meet your last girlfriend, spurring some of your greatest stories, and bringing out your worst dance moves but do you ever feel guilty about drinking a beer or two? Well there is really no need to feel guilty. Contrary to what you might expect, moderate beer consumption is actually good for you. That is a proven fact!

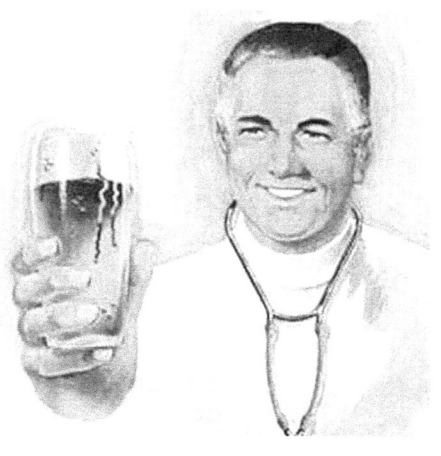

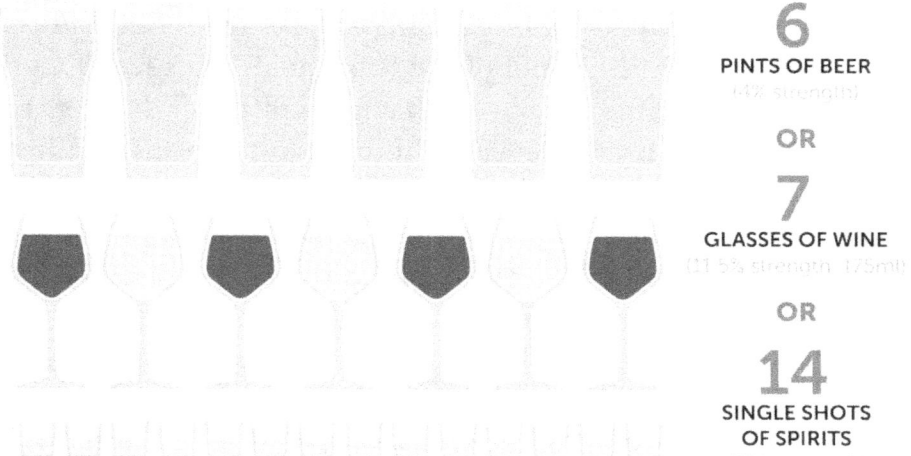

RECOMMENDED ALCOHOL CONSUMPTION
FOR MEN AND WOMEN

14 UNITS OF ALCOHOL A WEEK, WHICH IS:

6
PINTS OF BEER

OR

7
GLASSES OF WINE

OR

14
SINGLE SHOTS
OF SPIRITS

Science has shown that beer can bring many surprising health benefits even though it's usually perceived as unhealthy. Just remember, we're talking moderate consumption (one drink per day for women, and up to two for men), not all-night drinking sprees.

Below you will find some thirteen remarkable and surprising beer benefits that might change your perception and may even give beer a good name!

- **Reduced Risk of Heart Disease** - Wine usually gets all the credit as the drink that helps cut back your cardiovascular disease risk, but beer may be just as heart-healthy of a beverage. One eye-opening study involving 200,000 subjects conducted at Italy's Fondazion di Ricerca e Cura, found that people who drank a pint of beer daily had a 31% reduced chance of heart disease. This heart-protecting power of beer stems largely from beer's natural antioxidants called phenols. However, the study also showed risk of heart disease increased in people who consumed higher amounts of beer.
- **Protect Against Alzheimer's Disease** - Perhaps one of the most remarkable health benefits of beer is its ability to protect against Alzheimer's. Researchers at Loyola University Chicago Stritch School of Medicine analyzed several studies and came to the conclusion that moderate beer drinkers were 23% less likely to develop different forms of dementia and cognitive impairment, including Alzheimer's. The silicon content in beer is thought to protect the brain from the harmful effects of high amounts of aluminum in the body, which are one of the possible causes of Alzheimer's.
- **Lower Diabetes Risk** - Dutch researchers analyzed 38,000 male health professionals and found that when men who weren't big boozers began drinking moderately over 4 years, they were significantly less likely to be diagnosed with type 2

diabetes. In a 2011 Harvard study of about 40,000 middle-aged men, those who drank one to two beers daily had a 25% reduction in the risk of developing type 2 diabetes, confirming the Dutch research results. The alcohol content in beer increases insulin sensitivity, which helps prevent diabetes. Moreover, beer is a good source of soluble fiber that plays an important role in the healthy diet of people suffering from diabetes. Increased alcohol consumption over time didn't lower the risk in men who already had a couple drinks a day, so moderation is the key word here.

- **Say Goodbye to Kidney Stones** - Cheers to never having to pass a kidney stone again—or if you're lucky, ever. A study conducted in Finland established that moderate daily consumption of beer can reduce the risk of developing kidney stones by 40%. This health benefit is attributed to beer's high water content (about 93%) that helps flush harmful toxins out of the body and keep the kidneys working properly. Also, compounds in hops used in brewing help slow the release of calcium from bones, which in turn prevents build-up of lost calcium in the kidney in the form of stones.

- **Minimize Cancer Risk** - Beer contains an important antioxidant known as xanthohumol. Xanthohumol is known to have powerful anti-cancer properties that help fend off cancer-causing enzymes in the body. Specifically, moderate beer consumption helps prevent a certain chemical reaction that can lead to prostate cancer in men. Beer has also been shown to reduce the chances of getting breast cancer in women.

- **Reduce Levels of Cholesterol** - If you'd like an unorthodox method for cutting your cholesterol levels, indulging in moderate beer consumption may be the way to go. The barley used in brewing of beer contains a type of soluble fiber known as beta-glucans that has been shown to help in lowering cholesterol levels.

- Help Manage Blood Pressure - You may also be interested to know that beer can help manage blood pressure. That's according to a Harvard study that found that women aged 25 to 40 who drank beer moderately were significantly less likely to develop high blood pressure compared to women who drank wine or other alcoholic beverages.
- **Strengthen Your Bones** - Move over milk! Nasty breaks from drunken debauchery aside, a couple beers a day could actually strengthen your bones, according to a study at Tufts University. Beer contains decent levels of silicon, an element that is linked with bone health. One study conducted at Tufts in 2009 established that older individuals who drank one or two glasses of beer daily had higher bone density, and thus were less prone to fractures than those who did not enjoy a glass of beer or wine. However, the study also found that consuming more than two drinks increased risk of bone fractures.
- **Treat Dandruff** - Another interesting fact about beer is that it is considered one of the best natural treatments for dandruff. This particular health benefit of beer is attributed to its high yeast and vitamin B content levels. Just rinse your hair with a bottle of beer two to three times a week to get rid of dandruff and make your hair extra soft and shiny.
- **Reduce Stroke Risk** - Studies by the American Stroke Association have shown that people who drink moderate amounts of beer can cut their risk of strokes by – get this – a whopping 50% compared to non-drinkers. Researchers at Harvard School of Public Health explain that moderate amounts of beer daily will help prevent blood clots that block blood flow to the heart, neck and brain, which is a leading

cause of ischemic stroke. Also, when you drink beer moderately, your arteries become flexible and blood flow improves significantly. Remember the key to reaping these amazing health benefits of beer is moderate consumption. Overindulgence in beer and other alcoholic drinks can be disastrous to your health.

- **Fight Off Infection** - Having one or two drinks a day might boost your immune system and fight infections, according to an Oregon Health & Science University study. Scientists vaccinated monkeys against smallpox, then gave some of the primate's access to alcohol while others could drink sugar water. The monkeys who drank moderately had better vaccine responses than those who consumed the sweet stuff. But the animals that drank *heavily*—you may now imagine a totally tanked chimp—had less of a response to the vaccine than those who kept their habit under control.

- **Lower your blood pressure** - High blood pressure can be responsible for a range of health problems, but beer can lower your risk for hypertension, research suggests. In one study, Harvard researchers found that moderate beer drinkers are less likely to develop high blood pressure than those who sip wine or cocktails.

- **Better Vision through Beer** - We are not talking about beer goggles here! A Guinness a day could keep the eye doctor away. Canadian researchers found that one daily beer—especially a lager or stout—increases antioxidant activity that can stop cataracts from forming in the eyes. The kicker: The scientists found an opposite effect in participants who had three or more drinks a day.

HEALTH BENEFITS OF BEER

Aids in digestion

Promotes urination

Prevents anemia

Helps increase bone density

Lowers risk of kidney and gallstones

Caution: Drinking excessive amounts (addiction) is dangerous to health

Reduces stress and gives relief from insomnia

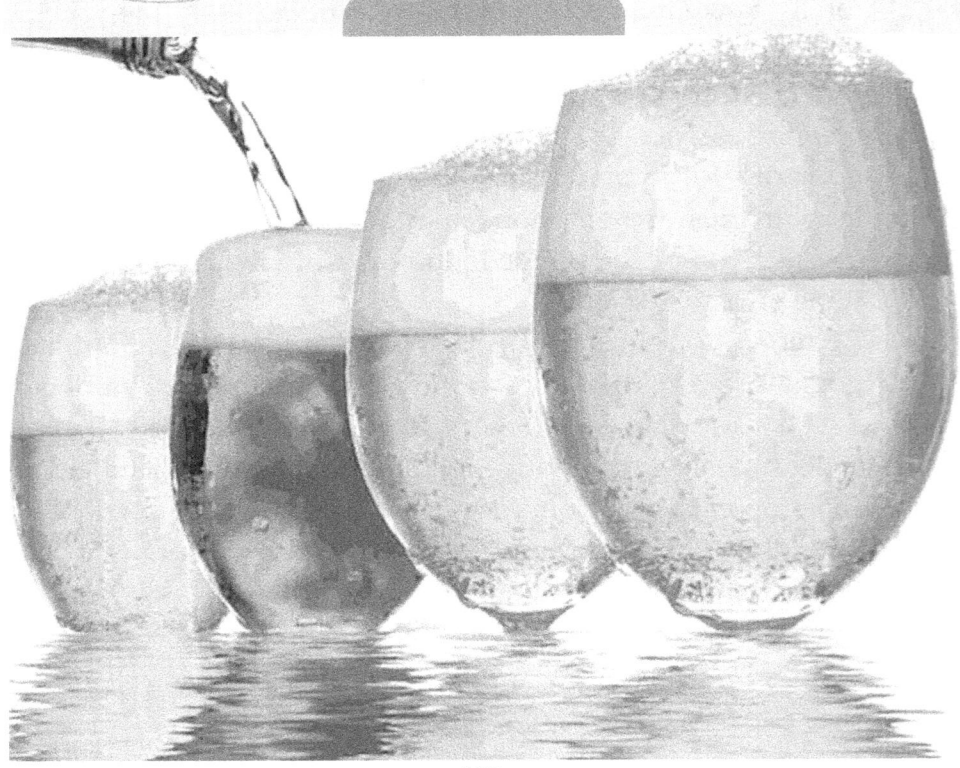

6 Conclusion

Look, while I could bow to convention and follow the "rules" of proper book layout and publishing, those that demand that in the conclusion I sum up all of the preceding chapters and answer any questions that may still remain in the minds of my readers, I would rather not.

Frankly I just don't want to do that. So, since I have never much been one for following all the "rules," I think I'll just approach this conclusion the way I want.

You see, I absolutely do not want to answer all of your questions with this book. In fact, I think that all of those so called, "all you need to know" books are ridiculous!

What I want to achieve with this work, what hope I have achieved is that I provided you with enough solid, scientific information that you are encouraged to start asking more questions about chocolate, wine, and beer; their history, their impact on mankind, and their possible impact on your health. I hope you do some additional research of your own! As for how I would sum up this book? Let me simply paraphrase something I said many times earlier in this work…

Too much of a good thing is not a good thing! Increased alcohol consumption over time will not lead to better health but could, in fact, ruin your health. What's more the same is true for the unchecked consumption of chocolate!

Moderation is the key word here!

I will leave you with just a few more bits of graphical information to consider:

This is what one drink looks like

According to the Dietary Guidelines for Americans, moderate drinking is up to one drink per day for women and up to two drinks per day for men. A standard drink contains 14 grams of pure alcohol.

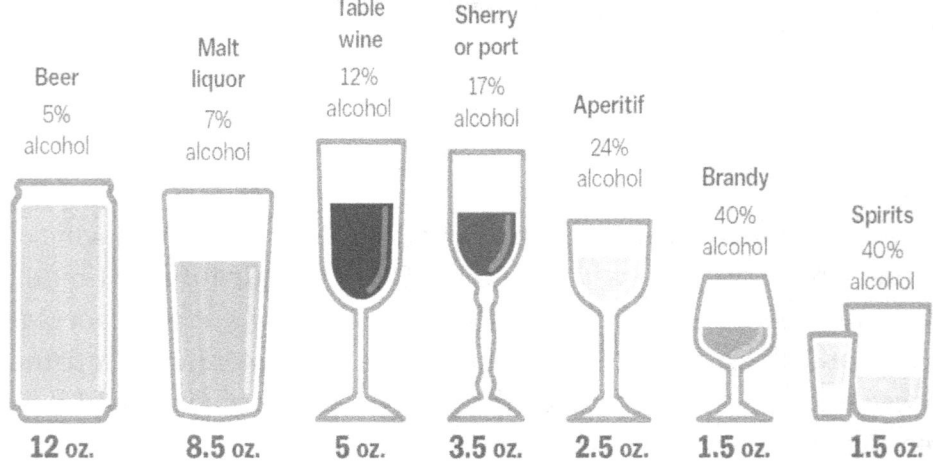

Measures are approximate, since different brands and beverages may vary in their actual alcohol content.

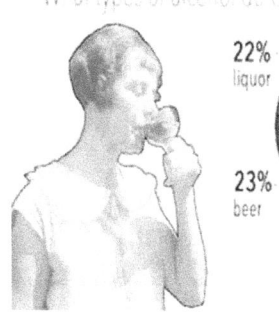

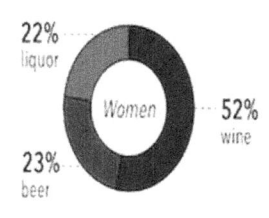

22%
liquor

Women

52%
wine

23%
beer

21%
liquor

Men

20%
wine

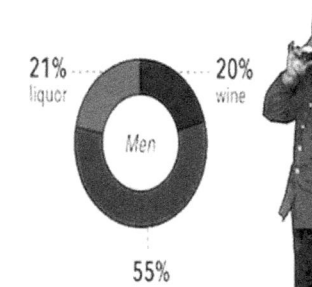

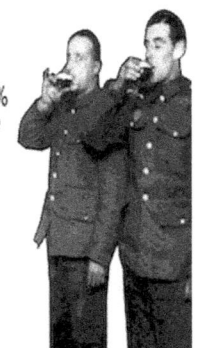

55%
beer

STANDARD-SIZED DRINK EQUIVALENTS
APPROXIMATE NUMBER OF STANDARD-SIZED DRINKS IN:

BEER or COOLER

12 oz.
~5% alcohol

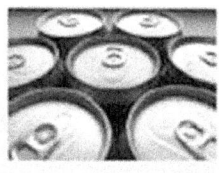

- 12 oz. = 1
- 16 oz. = 1.3
- 22 oz. = 2
- 40 oz. = 3.3

MALT LIQUOR

8–9 oz.
~7% alcohol

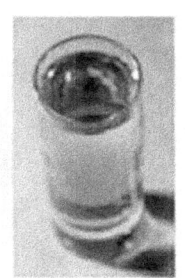

- 12 oz. = 1.5
- 16 oz. = 2
- 22 oz. = 2.5
- 40 oz. = 4.5

TABLE WINE

5 oz.
~12% alcohol

- a 750 mL (25 oz.) bottle = 5

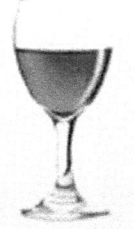

80-proof SPIRITS
(hard liquor)

1.5 oz.
~40% alcohol

- a mixed drink = 1 or more*
- a pint (16 oz.) = 11
- a fifth (25 oz.) = 17
- 1.75 L (59 oz.) = 39

Most popular varieties of table wine in the U.S. by market share

Chardonnay *21%*

Cabernet Sauvignon *12%*

Merlot *9%*

Pinot Grigio/Gris *8%*

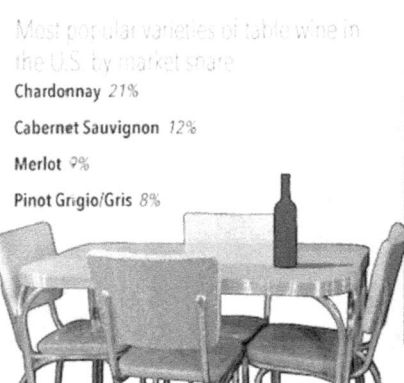

WINE SALES IN THE U.S.		
Year	Millions of 9-liter cases of wine	Total retail value
2008	313.8	$30 billion
2009	321.1	$28.7 billion
2010	329.7	$30 billion
2011	351.5	$32.9 billion
2012	360.1	$34.6 billion

WHICH IS HEALTHIER?

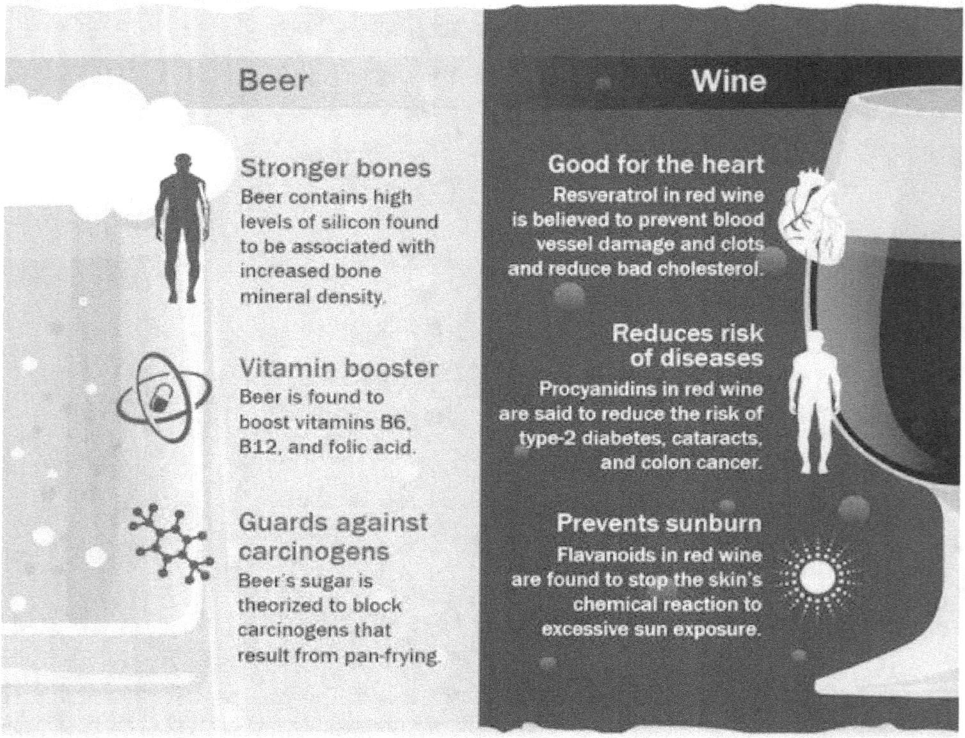

Beer

Stronger bones
Beer contains high levels of silicon found to be associated with increased bone mineral density.

Vitamin booster
Beer is found to boost vitamins B6, B12, and folic acid.

Guards against carcinogens
Beer's sugar is theorized to block carcinogens that result from pan-frying.

Wine

Good for the heart
Resveratrol in red wine is believed to prevent blood vessel damage and clots and reduce bad cholesterol.

Reduces risk of diseases
Procyanidins in red wine are said to reduce the risk of type-2 diabetes, cataracts, and colon cancer.

Prevents sunburn
Flavanoids in red wine are found to stop the skin's chemical reaction to excessive sun exposure.

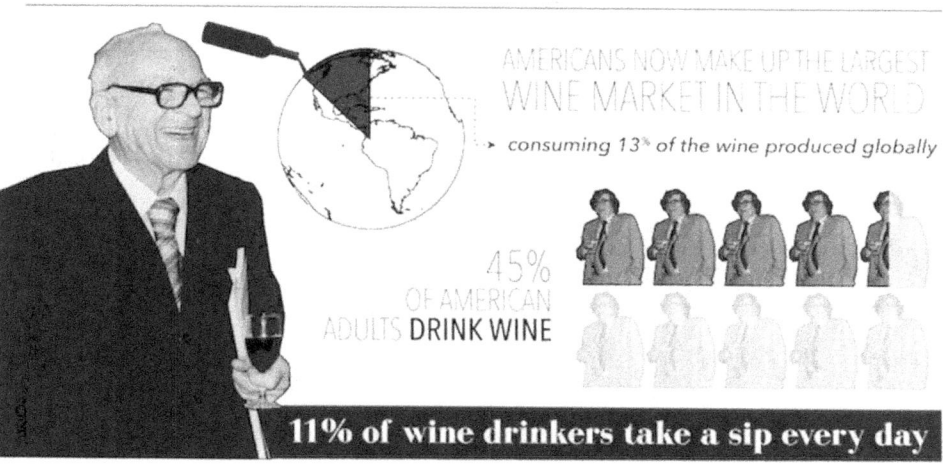

AMERICANS NOW MAKE UP THE LARGEST
WINE MARKET IN THE WORLD

consuming 13% of the wine produced globally

45%
OF AMERICAN
ADULTS DRINK WINE

11% of wine drinkers take a sip every day

WINE CONSUMPTION IN THE U.S.

Year	Wine per resident	Total gallons
2008	2.45 gals	746 million
2009	2.49 gals	763 million
2010	2.53 gals	784 million
2011	2.68 gals	836 million
2012	2.73 gals	856 million

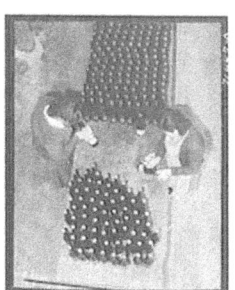

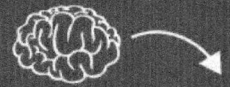

DRINKERS vs NON-DRINKERS

BRAIN function declines at a markedly faster rate in nondrinkers than in moderate drinkers.

MODERATE DRINKERS ARE:

50% less likely to have strokes.

30% less likely to develop type 2 diabetes.

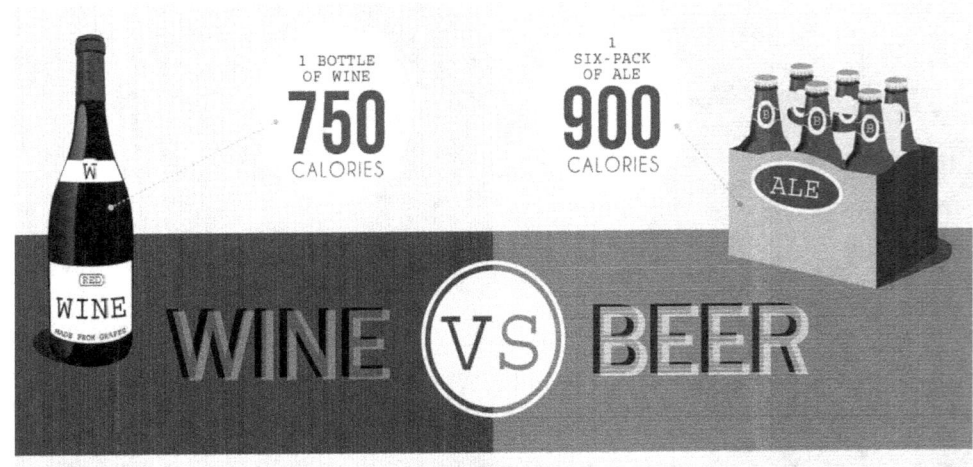

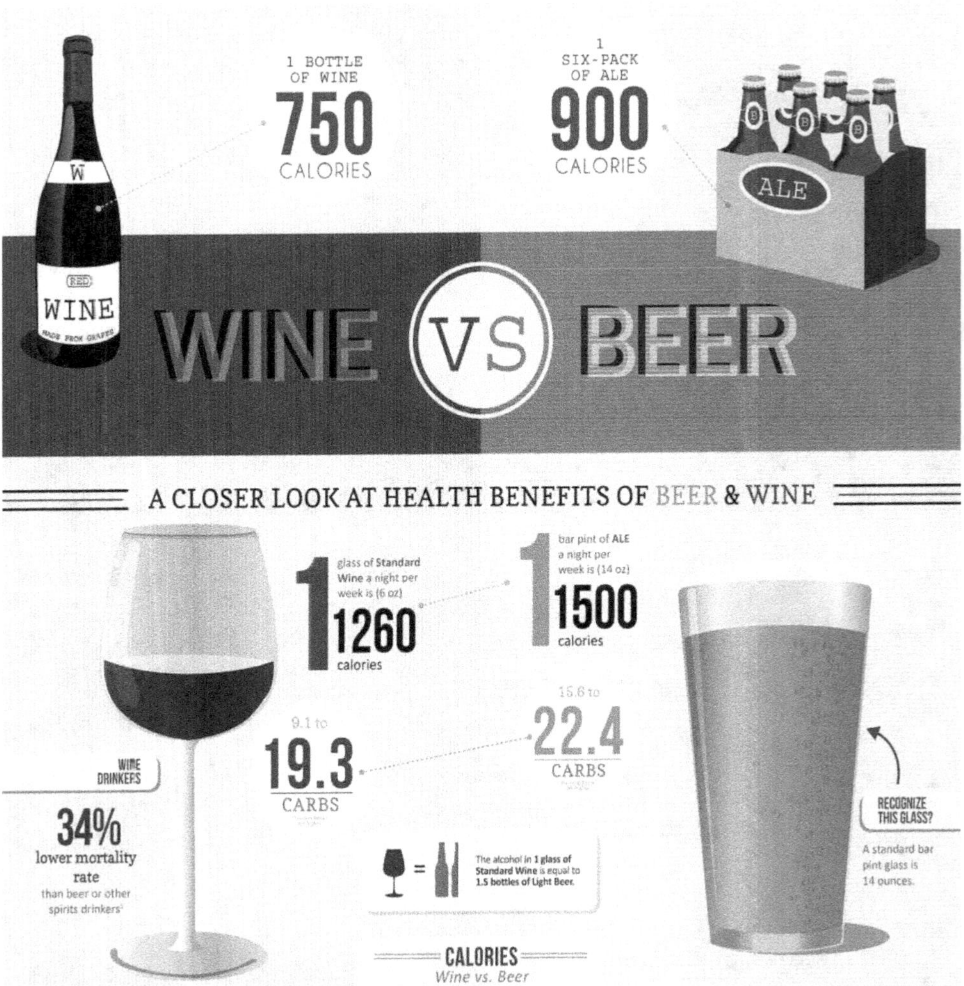

1 BOTTLE OF WINE
750 CALORIES

1 SIX-PACK OF ALE
900 CALORIES

WINE (VS) BEER

A CLOSER LOOK AT HEALTH BENEFITS OF BEER & WINE

1 glass of **Standard Wine** a night per week is (6 oz)
1260 calories

1 bar pint of **ALE** a night per week is (14 oz)
1500 calories

9.1 to
19.3 CARBS

15.6 to
22.4 CARBS

WINE DRINKERS

34% lower mortality rate than beer or other spirits drinkers[1]

🍷 = 🍺🍺 The alcohol in **1 glass** of **Standard Wine** is equal to **1.5 bottles of Light Beer.**

RECOGNIZE THIS GLASS?
A standard bar pint glass is 14 ounces.

CALORIES
Wine vs. Beer

LIGHT WHITE WINE (8-10% ABV) *Wines w/ less than 30 g/L residual sugar*	6 OZ	95 - 139 calories
CHAMPAGNE (12% ABV) *Brut Zero or Brut Nature*	8 OZ	125-160 calories
STANDARD WINE (12.5-13.5% ABV) *Dry Reds & Whites*	6 OZ	175 - 187 calories
HIGH ABV WINE (13.5-16% ABV) *Zinfandel, Shiraz, Chardonnay*	6 OZ	187 - 219 calories
DESSERT WINE (16-20% ABV) *Port, Sherry, Madeira*	3 OZ	220 - 260 calories

LIGHT BEER (3-4% ABV) *Amstel Light, Bud Light*	12 OZ 14 OZ	95 - 139 calories 110 - 162 calories
LAGER (4-5% ABV) *Bitburger, Coors*	12 OZ 14 OZ	140 - 191 calories 163 - 223 calories
ALE/IPA (5-6.5% ABV) *Fat Tire, Sierra Nevada*	12 OZ 14 OZ	163 - 228 calories 190 - 266 calories
BELGIUM (6.5-9.5% ABV) *Westmalle Tripel*	12 OZ	201 - 303 calories
IMPERIAL IPA (9-12% ABV) *Dogfish Head 90min. Ale*	12 OZ	260 - 360 calories